REMISSION QUEST

VIRGINIA ADAMS O'CONNELL

REMISSION QUEST

A Medical Sociologist Navigates Cancer

TEMPLE UNIVERSITY PRESS
Philadelphia • *Rome* • *Tokyo*

TEMPLE UNIVERSITY PRESS
Philadelphia, Pennsylvania 19122
tupress.temple.edu

Library of Congress Cataloging-in-Publication Data

Names: O'Connell, Virginia Adams author
Title: Remission quest : a medical sociologist navigates cancer / Virginia
 Adams O'Connell.
Description: Philadelphia : Temple University Press, 2025. | Includes
 bibliographical references and index. | Summary: "This book traces the
 author's journey through lymphoma diagnosis and treatment in light of
 her education and research in medical sociology. She uses her experience
 to illustrate how the field's predominate theories are experienced in
 practice and where the theories fall short"— Provided by publisher.
Identifiers: LCCN 2025003174 (print) | LCCN 2025003175 (ebook) | ISBN
 9781439926529 cloth | ISBN 9781439926536 paperback | ISBN 9781439926543
 pdf
Subjects: LCSH: O'Connell, Virginia Adams—Health |
 Lymphomas—Patients—Biography | Lymphomas—Patients—Social conditions
 | Medical sociologists—Biography
Classification: LCC RC280.L9 O36 2025 (print) | LCC RC280.L9 (ebook) |
 DDC 616.99/446—dc23/eng/20250425
LC record available at https://lccn.loc.gov/2025003174
LC ebook record available at https://lccn.loc.gov/2025003175

The manufacturer's authorized representative in the EU for product safety is Temple
University Rome, Via di San Sebastianello, 16, 00187 Rome RM, Italy (https://rome
.temple.edu/).
tempress@temple.edu

♾ The paper used in this publication meets the requirements of the American National
Standard for Information Sciences—Permanence of Paper for Printed Library Materials,
ANSI Z39.48–1992

Printed in the United States of America

9 8 7 6 5 4 3 2 1

This book is dedicated to all my Carcinomies.

CONTENTS

ACKNOWLEDGMENTS

I want to start by thanking three former professors who sparked my enchantment with the fields of sociology and anthropology—Wyatt MacGaffey, professor emeritus of anthropology, Haverford College; Renée C. Fox, professor emerita, University of Pennsylvania; and Charles L. Bosk, professor emeritus, University of Pennsylvania. Renée and Charles, both medical sociologists and bioethicists, passed away in 2020 and are dearly missed by their colleagues and by the medical communities they studied. All three were the finest mentors.

I want to thank Stephen A. O'Connell, my husband, who held my hand and heart during the agonizing period before the diagnosis and through treatment and who kept the household running smoothly, especially during my inpatient infusions; Hil O'Connell, my eldest, who cut my first pretreatment bob, made an incredible preadmission care package, and always made me laugh when needed; David O'Connell, my son, who, when I asked countless questions, helped me comprehend as best I could every medical procedure and every drug that was part of my treatment protocol; and Mary Kay Adams, my sister, an exemplary support person during both inpatient and outpatient infusions, master of the infusion-day picnic and needed distractions.

I want to thank my colleagues in the Department of Sociology and Anthropology at Moravian University who supported my taking a medical leave. While I appreciate all my colleagues, I especially want to thank Debra

Wetcher-Hendricks, my friend and colleague since I joined the Moravian faculty in 2008. Upon sharing my diagnosis, Deb gave me a very needed hug and then made sure without hesitation or complaint that all my classes were covered and my advisees supported.

And finally, thank you to CaringBridge, a no-cost, 501(c)(3) nonprofit online health platform that offers a way for patients to document a health journey, simplify care coordination, and connect caregivers with a supportive community. Using CaringBridge during my treatment provided me with a way to communicate with numerous family and friends near and far.

REMISSION QUEST

Introduction

Sociologist C. Wright Mills, in defining his concept of the sociological imagination, invites us all to experience the reality of our individual lives more fully by recognizing how our lives are influenced and shaped by the culture of the wider society, to see the relationship and interaction between the two.[1] Mills argues that only by considering how our experiences and behaviors are influenced by history and the structures of social institutions can we understand our circumstances. He also argues that theories are best understood in context, and that through the lens of the interaction between the individual and society, we can see the explicit and implicit, the intended and unintended consequences of the structures and functions of our social institutions. This wider view allows us all to see beyond the constraints of our own limited individual experiences and compels us to view issues from a broader context, to see our collective human experience more broadly.

Mills argues that using a sociological imagination is not limited to professors and students of sociology. All should use it since authentic self-understanding derives from understanding the circumstance of your life. He also argues that one of the advantages of this exercise is the ability to connect "personal troubles to public issues," possibly identifying paths for positive change, better outcomes, by changing aspects of our social institutions.

This book is the product of using my sociological imagination to share with you my story of being diagnosed with and treated for primary bone lymphoma in 2019. The experience expanded my sociological imagination—those theories of structures and their effects on individuals that I once studied as a sociologist observing the healthcare system and people navigating illness suddenly confronted my own reality. Throughout this account, I have woven together sociological theories with descriptions of my personal experiences to illustrate and enrich the sociological analysis of our medical institutions and of my own illness narrative. Those theories helped me make sense of my experience, yes, but so, too, did my experiences shine new light on those theories.

I am acutely aware that my cancer experience has been influenced by my wider society and by the circumstances of my past and present. My experience was affected by my being diagnosed in 2019 rather than prior to 1993, before CHOP and R-CHOP were effective treatments for lymphoma.[2] My experience of being diagnosed and treated in the United States rather than in another Western country resulted in my diagnosis being delayed for months due to my private insurer denying my primary physician's request for a PET scan, but also in my access to a preeminent medical institution, the Abramson Cancer Center at the University of Pennsylvania Hospital, where I received the best care currently available.

My experience, while in some ways uniquely mine, shares many traits with those of other cancer patients who were diagnosed and treated around the same time and who, like me, have yet to reach the coveted five-year post-treatment remission milestone. While our particular cancers, treatments, and prognoses vary based on our cancer types, we all face similar core questions about and challenges associated with our cancer experience. We have to face our own and the wider society's fear of cancer in America. We confront such fundamental questions as "Why me?" and "Why now?" We have to navigate the complex world of insurance and new financial burdens, including the potential loss of or temporary absence from employment. We must alter our lives to complete aggressive treatment protocols, and we have to manage the damage from surgery, radiation, and chemotherapy. We confront our mortality and wrestle with questions about the meaning of life, all while being exposed to harsh treatments that are hopefully killing our errant cells.

We navigate through elaborate medical systems, learning new sick roles, at the same time that we are trying to manage indescribable fear and fatigue. We are asked to be good compliant patients in medical settings, and we are asked by the wider society to be cheerful, grateful, and brave "warriors" who are battling our cancers. We are asked to do all of these things as we lose our hair and no longer recognize ourselves in the mirror. We try to maintain as many aspects of our pre-cancer lives as possible, especially since our existence itself might not be guaranteed.

We spend so much time in medical settings, learning new medical terms and a variety of practices to mitigate the side effects, that I might argue that the cancer patient should be awarded an education certificate or some academic credit at the end of the process. So much new knowledge!

In the midst of all of these challenges, the cancer patient can also experience forms of intimate interaction that most of us often do not get chances to experience as we navigate our busy modern lives. When receiving kind and competent medical care, the medical staff attends to our physical as well as to our emotional and spiritual needs. In the middle of the night in the hospital, the taking of vitals can be accompanied by an animated exchange about the challenges of parenting. The surgical nurse tightly holds your hand since he knows that the procedure you are about to have done is going to be more uncomfortable than you anticipate. The nurse administering your chemotherapy lets you cry for a few minutes before starting the infusion without judgment or impatience. The transporter in the hospital distracts you as he wheels you to a procedure by sharing all his favorite places in DELCO (Delaware County, where you both live). There are people you meet for the first and perhaps only time when you are at one of the lowest, most fraught places you have ever been, and they find ways to hold and support you.

There are also the intimate exchanges with fellow patients. The knowing nods as you walk the hallways, dragging your IV stands. The freedom to be brutally honest about how nauseous and exhausted you feel. The candid confession about how terrified you are about the upcoming scan. The spirited retelling of how and when your cancer was diagnosed. The ability to candidly laugh at the seeming absurdity of it all with others on the same journey who will not require that you do not talk about the pain or the challenges. We can shake our fists at the universe together.

The cancer patient embarks on a transformative and, I argue, perilous journey once the diagnosis is confirmed and treatment begins. In some ways, it is the beginning of an unending journey, as the fear of recurrence will remain, even after five years. My audience for this book is all of us—the patients, the caretakers, the medical staff, and the general public, as we all at the very least know someone at some point who has been diagnosed with cancer. In this complex narrative, I honor all the actors while suggesting ways we might improve all of our experiences, both in and out of medical settings. Because of my diagnosis, I joined a club of current and past patients that I never wanted or intended to join, but we can collectively work to make it the best club it can be.

1

Pursuing the Diagnosis

The first time the pain in my right arm and shoulder captured my full attention was on Thursday, February 8, 2019, on my morning drive to Moravian University in Bethlehem, Pennsylvania. To avoid commuter traffic, I leave my home in Swarthmore by 5:45 A.M. on the days that I commute. Much later than that and I risk hitting significant traffic on Route 476 (the Northeast Extension) before Exit 20 (Plymouth Meeting) and then face another possible significant delay on Route 22, which takes me east to Bethlehem once I get off Route 476 at Exit 56. Up until the ride that morning, any discomfort that I had felt in my right arm and shoulder could be readily explained by a particularly robust game of squash, which at the time I was playing at least twice a week. But on that very dark and chilly morning, the pain was unusually achy and distracting. I remember periodically trying to stretch my shoulder and rotate it a bit as I was driving, but the dull ache continued.

Once I got to my office, I took some ibuprofen, and I also decided that between classes, I would ice my shoulder with a makeshift ice pack I made by filling about halfway a water bottle that I had in the communal refrigerator and putting it in the freezer. The ibuprofen and the ice together provided some temporary relief.

On that particular Thursday, instead of commuting home, I was staying overnight in Bethlehem at a local hotel, as I was meeting a friend of mine, a high-school teacher, for dinner in Bethlehem. After dinner, we planned on visiting an art exhibit on Moravian's campus. I also had a meeting scheduled for the next morning on campus.

I do not tend to sleep well in hotel rooms, but on this evening, it was not the unfamiliarity of the room and the lack of my favorite pillow that were interfering with my sleep so much as the increasing pain in my right shoulder. I took two ibuprofen tablets and concocted a pillow support for my arm, and still I could not get comfortable. After a very fitful evening, I headed back to campus. Once in my office, I tried icing my shoulder again, having left the water bottle in the freezer. I again got some temporary relief, but my level of concern was rising. I hated to think that I had an injury that might need medical attention and cause me to miss my next squash game!

I drove home after my meeting, now taking ibuprofen as often as I could while still following the bottle's instructions. I was exhausted by the time I got home due to my lack of sleep the night before. My husband had a dinner meeting and a lecture to attend, so I ordered some Chinese takeout and headed to bed early.

My husband got home around 9:30 P.M. that night, and I awoke as our two dogs stirred when they heard him come in. As I tried to roll over, the pain in my shoulder was suddenly unbearable. I got up out of bed and howled. My husband came running up the stairs, asking if I was okay, and I stood there in the middle of the bedroom, feeling as though I might black out, the pain was so intense. I tried to calm down. I started focusing on my breathing. The pain dissipated a bit, but my arm now hung loosely at my side, as I was scared to move it in case the pain returned. In less than forty-eight hours, I went from thinking, "Well, that is an annoying ache" to making plans to go to the emergency room.

We headed to the Crozer-Chester Medical Center in Chester, Pennsylvania. I was hesitant to go at first since it was a Friday night, and Friday nights in emergency rooms tend to be filled with "true" emergencies—car accident victims, for example. At first, I felt an obligation to try to "tough it out" until the next morning, so that the attention of the emergency room staff would be spent on patients whose lives needed immediate saving, but my husband convinced me that I needed to be checked and, at the very least, needed some pain relief, so we headed over. The ER at Crozer, luckily for us, was not crowded when we arrived. It was now about 11:00 P.M., and it was not long before we were taken back to a bay. The attending physician who saw me had a personable demeanor that I greatly appreciated, especially given how late it was. I even apologized for being there, but he did not for a moment make me feel as though I were wasting anyone's time or resources. After reviewing my vitals and taking my history, he sent me for some X-rays to get a better view of what was happening with my shoulder. The X-rays showed some "mild degenerative change of the acromioclavicular joint with spurring," but no fracture or dislocation. Based on the X-rays and my symptoms, I was diagnosed with a frozen shoulder. Also known as adhesive capsulitis, frozen shoulder results from a thickening of the shoulder capsule, the connective tissue that holds the humerus in place in the shoulder joint.[1] I presented with classic symptoms: (1) It most commonly affects people between the ages of forty and sixty (I was then fifty-five), (2) it occurs more often in women, and (3) pain can start off slowly but then be experienced as severe pain, rendering the individual unable to move the shoulder. The suggested intervention that evening (now early morning) was a joint injection of an anesthetic (lidocaine) mixed with a steroid (Kenalog). The attending did a masterful job with the joint injection. I was sent home with a prescription for some oral steroids, told to use over-the-counter pain relief if needed, and had instructions to continue icing the shoulder and a recommendation to make an appointment with an orthopedist as soon as possible.

I was able to make an appointment with an orthopedist for February 13, which I thought was very lucky—just a few days! The shoulder was still somewhat uncomfortable, but I definitely felt better after the shot and on the oral steroids. It was still somewhat painful to move my right arm much, but I was not concerned—I took comfort in thinking that was normal for a frozen shoulder. I suspected that following some rest and the completion of the oral steroids, I would begin a course of treatment with a physical therapist to help unfreeze the shoulder.

My appointment with the orthopedist on February 13 was very short, as he wanted me to get an MRI to take a closer look at the shoulder to assess whether there was an injury that the X-ray could not detect. The office staff helped me get an MRI appointment for that afternoon. I had a follow-up appointment to review the MRI scheduled for February 20.

The morning of February 20, I awoke with acute gastroenteritis. I called the office to cancel the appointment, promising to call them back to reschedule as soon as I could access my calendar. I called the next day and scheduled a new appointment for February 26.

I recall being annoyed on the morning of February 26. I did not want to head back to the orthopedist's office. I wished that he could have just called me with the MRI results and prescribed some physical therapy. I had a ton of errands I needed to do that day since I was not commuting to Bethlehem. I had to go to the grocery store and the post office, get the dogs out for a walk, and make some phone calls.

As soon as I was brought back to the exam room, I sensed that something was very amiss. At my previous appointment, a scribe had been in the room with us. The same scribe entered the room before the doctor, and he would not make eye contact with me. He nervously adjusted his laptop on his rolling cart. I could not understand why he would not look at me.

A few moments later, the doctor came into the room. During our previous meeting, he had been almost overly garrulous, conducting my initial exam with swagger. Upon entering the room now, his face was void of emotion. In his hand were the results of my MRI. He stretched out his arm to hand me the report and said, "You have cancer."

I admit how clichéd this sounds, but time seemed to stop for a moment. Immediately, the scribe's reluctance to look at me made sense. He knew that this news was coming. I thought of all the errands I had to do that day. I thought about how I was only fifty-five years old, how healthy I had felt before the morning of February 8, how I did not have time for this, and when time resumed, I responded to the news with a harrowing laugh. This could not be happening.

I asked, "What kind of cancer?" They had no idea. I sat, shaking my head. The doctor offered to call my husband, a professor of economics, who was at work at Swarthmore College, just a few miles from the doctor's office. At first, I said not to bother him, but the doctor insisted. Everyone left me in the exam room, and I started to cry.

I looked at the MRI report: "There is abnormal signal throughout the near complete proximal humerus involving the humeral head and neck, as well as the visible proximal shaft, as demonstrated by diffuse increased T2 and severely low T1 signal, with the exception of a small portion of the humeral head. There is additionally diffuse periosteal edema. Similar foci of signal abnormality are present within the glenoid and in the coracoid process. These findings are in keeping with osseous malignancy. These findings are suspicious for metastatic disease. There is no pathologic fracture."

I am a sociologist, not a health professional or a natural scientist. I did start off college as a chemistry major, and I am a medical sociologist, so I have always loved science. I recognized a good portion of these words, but certainly not all. The cancer was in my bone (osseous malignancy), but it was likely a cancer that had spread from somewhere else (metastatic). The pain I was feeling was not in my shoulder; it was emanating from my humerus.

When my husband got to the office, the doctor came back into the exam room. I asked whether the MRI findings were accurate and what kind of cancer it was most likely to be. He said that it was very likely the findings were accurate and that if he had to guess, given that it had spread to my arm, it was breast cancer. Although any cancer can spread to the bones, the most likely to are breast, kidney, lung, lymphoma, multiple myeloma, prostate, and thyroid.[2] I could immediately rule out prostate! Next step—find the source.

My husband and I headed home—in separate cars, unfortunately. As soon as I got in the door, I got on the phone to contact my internist. I also started calling to see whether I could get a mammogram as soon as possible. I am certain that even though I was trying to remain calm while making these calls, I likely sounded quite desperate, as the Crozer-Chester breast imaging center squeezed me into their schedule the next day, February 27. The process had begun.

I spent the rest of the afternoon on February 26 reading medical journal articles that I could only fractionally comprehend, with such titles as "Incidence and Evaluation of Incidental Abnormal Bone Marrow Signal on Magnetic Resonance Imaging."[3] I desperately searched for information that could help relieve my anxiety and read "Not Everything That Is Hot on a Staging Bone Scan Is Malignant: A Pictorial Review of Benign Causes of Increased Isotope Uptake" multiple times.[4] We decided not to tell anyone—not our children or our siblings—about this news, as we wanted to spare them from imagining possible worst-case scenarios until we had more information and a potential type of cancer. Not sharing the information was brutally hard, but I took comfort in knowing that we already had the next appointment. Soon, I thought, we would know more about what we were facing.

Little did I know that afternoon that I would not get a confirmed diagnosis of lymphoma until early June—five months after that morning drive in February. We began the long process of "rule out the most likely cancers," a process that I came to experience as a frantic game of whack-a-mole. Over the weeks and months, each new test ruled out one cancer but did not reveal the source. Each test result provided some comfort but also increased my frustration and fear. I could not treat the cancer until I knew which cancer I had. My mind raced when I imagined possible rapid progression of an untreated disease. But with each negative test result, I allowed myself, even for a moment, to hope that maybe, just maybe, the original MRI report was a mistake.

Breast

My mammogram was performed on February 27. The attending radiologist was kind enough to meet with me and perform an ultrasound in addition to the mammogram since the MRI had also indicated a slightly enlarged lymph node in my armpit. She said that nothing she was seeing at this point, including the lymph node, concerned her. I got the formal results of the mammogram on March 1: "The result of your diagnostic mammogram on 02/27/2019 appears to be normal." One down.

Bloodwork and Orders for CT Scans

My primary care physician saw me later in the afternoon on February 27 and ordered comprehensive blood work since some blood tests can give insight into the presence of cancer and possible cancer types. He also ordered CT scans of my chest and abdomen/pelvis, looking for possible evidence of lung, liver, ovarian, and colon cancer. All my blood results looked good and were in the normal range!

CT Scans

The CT scans were done on March 5, and the results were unremarkable. They found a few mildly enlarged lymph nodes, some thickening of the walls of my colon, and a small hiatal hernia (my stomach was sitting a bit high). But here is what looked normal: my lungs (except for some very minor scarring), heart, liver, pancreas, spleen, adrenal glands, kidneys and ureters, bladder, and pelvic organs (except for one fibroid). Regarding my bones, the results also indicated that I had "degenerative changes of the thoracic spine"—basically, very minor disc slippage. My first thought upon reading my bone result was that I did not need to know that!

The report concluded by recommending that I follow up the scan with a colonoscopy.

Appointments

My colonoscopy was scheduled for March 20, so I did now have some time to wait between tests. Between the CT scan and the colonoscopy, I underwent a scan of my thyroid that showed nothing remarkable (another cancer crossed off the list). In retrospect, I was fortunate to be able to schedule these tests as quickly as I did since in the absence of my persistence and professional familiarity with communicating with medical facilities and personnel as a medical sociologist, I would have likely had to wait weeks for an opening. I often had to "call around" to different offices and facilities. I was driven to aggressively pursue these appointments since the relief I had gotten from the original injection of the anesthetic and steroids in my shoulder was quickly fading, and the pain was rapidly increasing.

Colonoscopy

The final results of the colonoscopy were received on March 26 and were unremarkable. The doctor biopsied some inflamed tissue (the report found nothing suspicious) and found diverticulosis in my entire colon (again, since I had no symptoms or discomfort, I did not need to know this!), but the final assessment was that everything looked clear. The office staff asked me whether I wanted to pursue testing for possible Crohn's disease, a suggestion I quickly rejected. One major health issue at a time!

PET Scan

Since all the tests thus far had failed to find the source of the cancer, my primary care physician ordered a PET scan. "PET scans use a radioactive tracer to show how an organ is functioning in real time. PET scan images can detect cellular changes in organs and tissues earlier than CT and MRI scans."[5] Since my pain was increasing, we both knew that we had to continue the search and that the cancer had been thus far undetectable with the tests I had already had.

I had a PPO plan through my insurance provider that thus far had approved all my appointments and tests. My doctor requested the PET scan on March 25. On March 28, I received a letter informing me that the request was denied: "Based on our review, this service or supply is not approved because it does not satisfy the criteria for establishing medical necessity and appropriateness. . . . Your records do not describe results of a biopsy that support the need for further imaging." We were running out of tests, and I feared that we were running out of time.

Bone Scan Plan

My primary care physician decided to order a bone scan since although my insurance provider would not cover the cost of a PET scan, it would cover a bone scan. Bone scans and PET scans use radioactive tracers that are picked up by cells that are injured and repairing (such as bruised or broken bones) or by cells that are rapidly dividing (such as cancer cells). Although the basic technology is similar, the costs are quite different. The average national cost of a bone scan in the United States is $1,255, while the cost of a PET scan is $4,637.[6] PET scans are almost four times as expensive.

If the bone scan continued to show significant activity in the humerus, then perhaps a bone biopsy was in order. The earliest I could schedule the bone scan was April 15.

More waiting.

Increasing Pain

During these many weeks, I was still teaching my courses at Moravian University. By this point, the pain in my right arm/shoulder was becoming intolerable, and I was taking ibuprofen and acetaminophen around the clock. It was extremely uncomfortable to move my right arm, so driving and working on the computer became increasingly hard. I could no longer raise my right arm to write on the chalk- and whiteboards at work (I am right-handed), so I was using my left hand whenever I could write or draw legibly, such as when mapping a scatterplot in my advanced methods class. I quickly adapted to using my left hand to operate my computer mouse. Even the most basic personal grooming activities were becoming hard. I could not raise my right arm to brush my hair and adapted to imperfectly brushing with my left.

During the day, teaching and interacting with my colleagues and students helped keep my anxiety at bay and distract me from the pain, but the evenings were torturous. I could not get relief. Lying as flat as possible in the bathtub in very hot water provided relief for about fifteen minutes. I ended up sleeping upright in a chair each night, as lying down was impossible. One of my dogs, a small Pomeranian mix (that actually looks like a Jack Russell) named Bowie, undeniably knew that something was wrong. Since the original "injury," he would not leave my side. For months, he slept on my lap in whatever chair was my makeshift "bed" for that night. I started calling him my "nursey." I tried using a stronger pain relief medication (tramadol) since I was becoming increasingly sleep-deprived, but the tramadol made me feel too disoriented and, even on a very low dose, made me vomit, so I went back to relying on over-the-counter pain relievers.

Bone Scan Results

The bone scan results were sent to my doctor by the end of the day on April 15, and the image showed my humerus lighting up like a Christmas tree. Something remained unquestionably wrong; the MRI report was not a mistake. I called my primary care physician and asked whether we could please now request a bone biopsy, as I suspected that this test was the only way we were going to solve this diagnostic puzzle. He called a number of local orthopedic surgeon colleagues and was having trouble finding someone who could fit me in their schedule as soon as possible, but he ended up contacting an orthopedic surgeon specializing in bone cancers at the University of Pennsylvania Abramson Cancer Center, and she agreed to see me and do the biopsy if she believed that it was warranted. Her earliest availability was May 20. More waiting ahead.

Bone Biopsy

At the appointment on May 20, the orthopedist agreed to schedule a bone biopsy and sent me for an X-ray to see how much the humerus might have changed since my original X-ray in the ER back in February. She noted that often when cancer has spread to the bones, the bones can take on a "Swiss cheese" appearance. Bizarrely, even after so many months between pictures, the X-ray still looked "good," and she was encouraged. She did note "patchy areas of subtle lucency in the proximal right humerus [that] correspond[ed] to the areas of abnormal marrow seen on prior MRI."

The biopsy was scheduled for May 24. I was extremely grateful that the wait was so short. Soon, I kept reminding myself. Soon, we would know.

I was very nervous about the procedure, but it went smoothly. As I was waking up from the anesthesia, I overheard an orthopedic surgeon resident proudly telling the team that she had taken very good samples. I gratefully sighed. I knew that it would take some time to get the pathology report, but I was confident that we would finally have a clear diagnosis.

The Biopsy Report

A little over a week after my biopsy, my husband was scheduled to travel to Nairobi, Kenya, to attend a biannual workshop sponsored by the African Economic Research Consortium, a group with which he has worked his entire professional career. I was a bit anxious about his leaving since I had not gotten the biopsy results yet, but we had been trying to maintain as normal a routine as we could since that first ER visit, and he regularly made this trip. It did not seem to make sense for him not to travel, as we were unsure of when we would hear from the orthopedist. He was scheduled to leave on June 2 and would be returning on the afternoon of June 6.

On June 3, the orthopedist called. She said that the first analysis of my samples did not find cancer cells. The pathologist did find significant necrosis (dead cells), but he was perplexed as to the cause. I was simultaneously relieved and annoyed, as I was left again with no answer. She said that she would consult with my primary care physician and have him call me when they had a plan on next steps.

In the early afternoon on June 6, I had been on a work call and missed a call from the orthopedist. She left a voicemail message asking me to call her back. My heart leapt into my throat. As I finished dialing, I saw a cab pull up in front of my house: My husband was home from his trip. My call was transferred to the doctor, and with the dogs barking in excitement at my husband's return, I took my phone into the first-floor bathroom so I could hear the call. She told me that I had lymphoma—specifically, primary bone lymphoma.

The pathologist had called her back on June 5. He had been so perplexed by the initial analysis of my samples that he could not sleep the night of June 3 and had decided to redo the tests on my samples, which is when he finally found it: "This unusual spindle-cell shaped clone represents a variant of diffuse large B cell lymphoma." She was incredibly kind as she delivered the news. She said that if they had to find something, lymphoma was one of the more manageable diagnoses. She would be sharing all her findings with the oncology team at Penn, and someone would be in touch to schedule a PET scan and my first meeting with an oncologist. I finally qualified for a PET scan.

I thanked her for her kindness and told her to send a very special thank you to the pathologist for going back to the samples, and then I started to weep. I had my diagnosis, and soon I would have a plan of action.

I stepped out of the bathroom and found my husband, still in his coat, standing in the kitchen. I am sure that by the look on my face, I did not have to say anything, but as he took me into his arms, I said, "It's lymphoma."

That afternoon, I made calls to my children and to my sister. And then I spent some time online researching primary bone lymphoma, "a rare neoplasm of malignant lymphoid cells presenting with one or more bone lesions without nodal or other extranodal involvement. It accounts for approximately 1% of all lymphomas and 7% of malignant primary bone tumors."[7] Up until the phone call from the orthopedist, I had held some glimmer of hope that I could dodge a bullet, that the original MRI report had been mistaken. I now had to transfer the remaining hope toward a successful treatment experience.

PET Scan and First Oncology Appointment

With the diagnosis confirmed, a new reality began. My PET scan was scheduled for the morning of June 12. I already had a vet appointment for my dogs on June 11 and carpet cleaners coming on the afternoon of June 12 (I have plans, commitments, errands to run, I do not have time for this). My first oncology appointment was on June 13, and I had some organizing to do for the engagement party we were hosting for my eldest, their partner, and our friends and family on that Saturday, June 15, in our backyard.

At my oncology appointment, my physician showed me my PET scan. He showed how my humerus was brightly lit and how I also had bright spots on my femurs and both sides of my hip bones—the cancer had spread. It was therefore now Stage 4. He shared information about what to expect from the treatment protocol and said that I had to complete a few more tests before the first infusion—an echocardiogram (June 18), an MRI of my head (June 20), and the placement of a port (also June 20). My first infusion would be on June 21.

The perilous transition began.

Adopting the Sick Role and
Interpreting the Prognosis

Sick Role Imperatives

Talcott Parsons, one of the first medical sociologists, proposes an analytical framework to help examine the roles people adopt when they are sick. Since it is in society's interest to have ill members get well as soon as possible, Parsons argues that part of the responsibility we feel to be functioning members of society when we are ill is to seek legitimate medical care and to do everything possible to resume our normative roles.[1] In many medical systems, and particularly in healthcare systems in the United States, multiple structural barriers hinder our ability to seek confirmation of illness and, eventually, treatment. Lack of insurance or limited insurance coverage creates barriers to access and ability to pay for care. In January 2022, 12.5% of non-elderly adults in the United States were uninsured, with another 43% underinsured despite the increased access to insurance provided by the Affordable Care Act.[2] A 2009 study conducted by researchers at Harvard Medical School estimated that about forty-five thousand Americans die every year as a direct result of not having health insurance coverage.[3] A Gallup poll from 2019 found that 25% of Americans say that they or their family had put off treatment for a serious medical condition during the past year because of the cost.[4] A study published in 2018 found that one in seven uninsured patients could not make a primary care appointment if they could not show that they could pay the full cash amount for the visit.[5] And even for those who manage to get appointments, the uninsured are at significantly greater risk for delaying or not filling their prescriptions, being diagnosed at later stages of disease, and having higher mortality rates than people with insurance.[6,7,8]

Distance to medical facilities, a problem rural communities increasingly face as healthcare systems merge due to financial pressures, is also a significant hurdle and affects care outcomes.[9,10] These numerous and daunting financial and structural barriers create a tension between our recognition of the expectations placed upon us to get better and the ability to fulfill them. About 58% of all patients report some delay in accessing care due to any combination of these structural and financial constraints.[11]

The tension between the obligation demanded by Parsons's sick role to seek legitimate medical care and to do everything possible to get better and resume our normative roles and the barriers to accessing said care calls to mind the similarly impossible task Americans are told throughout their lives—"pull yourself up by your bootstraps." While the phrase was first interpreted in the 1800s as sarcastic advice since by the laws of physics, this act is impossible, by the 1970s, this phrase had become deeply ingrained in American culture and vernacular and over the years has come to be reinterpreted to mean improving oneself though one's individual efforts, a fundamental American value.[12] Whatever positive impact an inspirational call to action might have on the hearer, the call is cruel to make to the person who cannot possibly act. As Martin Luther King Jr. notes in a 1968 address, "It's alright to tell a man to lift himself by his own bootstraps, but it is a cruel jest to say to a bootless man that he ought to lift himself by his own bootstraps."[13] Holding patients accountable for accessing care and following treatment protocols when the system places so many obstacles in their way is a cruel jest.

It was difficult enough for me to navigate the system with the advantages of being employed, insured, educated, and socialized to communicate with the medical system. Even with these advantages, I lost valuable time before arriving at a treatment plan—and struggled to fill the roles I expected from myself in daily life. Imagine if I had not had those advantages.

Temptation of Denial

Despite the pressure to seek a diagnosis and care, in the beginning of an illness experience, when symptoms first appear, a subset of patients initially avoid seeking medical care, even if they have insurance. This phenomenon has been documented in many studies. It is different from the structural and financial barriers discussed earlier and from a delayed diagnosis, where a patient is actively seeking care, but the diagnosis is delayed. About 33% of all patients (those with and without insurance) avoid care because of unfavorable evaluations of seeking medical care, such as factors related to physicians and healthcare organizations, including low trust of doctors and/or a previous unpleasant experience. About 12% of insured patients delay because they expect their illness or symptoms to improve over time without intervention. About 25% delay because they fear that they have a serious illness.[5,11,14] You can see in my story how I confronted the reality of these temptations, such as when I considered not going to the emergency room on a busy Friday night. Why do people delay?

These avoidance behaviors are correlated with some well-documented demographics. A first hurdle is that an individual must recognize that they are sick. As noted previously, this process involves in part an assessment of limitation—can I continue to function? Because throughout our life course, as our expectations for functioning change due to age, energy demands, and shifting responsibilities, we can be more or less concerned about the same initial symptoms. The aches and pains that might be common for a fifty-five-year-old would be quite disconcerting for a twenty-five-year-old! Delay may be a consequence of our changing expectations for how we are supposed to feel, what symptoms might just be the inevitable impacts of aging. Intolerable pain or dysfunction is a common first hurdle we often fail to clear to seek medical care.

In anthropologist Mark Zborowski's classic 1969 work, *People in Pain*, he argues that how we interpret pain, and therefore assess how seriously we are ill, is significantly influenced by the cultures in which we are socialized.[15] Among the patients he studied, Jewish and Italian patients displayed emotional responses to pain far greater than those expressed by "old" American, Protestant patients. Medical settings, based on their own structures and cultures, define the expected and acceptable displays of pain, labeling those who are "overly" expressive as disruptive or, at worst, mentally unstable. A pervasive cultural preference for the "stiff upper lip," the display of fortitude and stoicism in the face of pain and other disruptive symptoms, contributes to the delay in seeking care and treatment in the United States. As I discuss later, this expectation complicates women's experiences in healthcare settings.

Race has also been shown to have a significant impact on the likelihood of experiencing pain, on the interpretation of pain, on the delay in seeking treatment, and in the eventual treatment prescribed. In studies investigating people over the age of fifty, 27% of African Americans and 28% of Hispanics reported having severe pain most of the time, compared to only 17% of non-Hispanic White people.[16] This difference is partly explained by the higher likelihood of minorities in the United States having on average poorer health insurance and fewer structural resources, such as education, resulting in a greater likelihood of experiencing chronic disease and distress, factors that increase the likelihood of experiencing severe pain.[17] While studies suggest that different racial groups do not rate pain intensity differently, African Americans do report pain as a more unpleasant sensation than do other groups at the same intensity.[18] However, African American subjects are significantly more likely to underreport pain unpleasantness in clinical settings, especially in the presence of physicians, suggesting particular discomfort with being honest about their pain experiences in this setting.[17] But even when we hold the pain discomfort level constant (remembering that African Americans are more likely to underreport), African American and Hispanic patients are less likely to receive pain medication, or they receive lower doses of pain medication.[18] All of these studies suggest that clinicians incorrectly believe that African American and Hispanic patients are exaggerating their pain experiences and are more likely to abuse pain medications than are their White counterparts, a conclusion with no support since White people are significantly more likely to misuse. Variations in treatment are based on misconceptions.[19] Considering minorities' greater share of structural and financial burdens to access care along with the disparate and undertreatment they receive when they do access care, their greater likelihood of delaying care becomes increasingly explicable.

The correlation of sex with frequency and expediency of accessing care is a more complex picture. Women continue to have longer life expectancies in the United States. In 2020, the average life expectancy of the U.S. population was 77.8 years, with a female life expectancy of 80.5 compared to the men's 75.1.[20] Women's longer life expectancy is in part due to basic biology, separate from medical care. Scientists believe that the higher levels of the hormone estrogen in women combat such conditions as heart disease by helping reduce circulatory levels of harmful cholesterol. Women are also thought to have stronger immune systems than men.[21] There are also behavioral factors, such as men's greater propensity to engage in risky and violent behaviors, pursue more dangerous work, and smoke and drink to excess. Some of these behaviors result from cultural expectations for men to publicly display their masculinity, leading them to be more likely to die of accidents, violence, and chronic conditions.[22,23]

Beyond these biological and behavioral factors, could women's longer life expectancy result from better and more frequent access to medical care? A 2001 report from the Centers for Disease Control and Prevention (CDC) found that women were 33% more likely than men to visit a doctor, averaging 4.6 visits a year compared to men's 3.8.[24] But we cannot assume that these visits are equally effective in diagnosing and treating illness; the greater number of visits might be the product of gender bias in healthcare settings. Women have to make more visits before they have their health concerns adequately addressed.

Gender bias against women in all realms of life is well documented. A 2020 United Nations report found that close to 90% of all men and women across the globe hold prejudiced views against women, helping explain women's significant global underrepresentation in positions of power (government and industry) and their pay disparity.[25] And this bias is expressed in various ways in healthcare settings.

When faced with financial constraints, women are significantly more likely than men to delay treatment, suggesting a greater deprioritizing of their care by the individual woman and her family. In 2017, Gallup found that 37% of women compared to 22% of men put off treatment due to cost, even when 63% of those who delayed treatment reported that their condition was very or somewhat serious.[26] This financial sacrifice is one of the first examples of women's differential access to care.

A 2018 extensive review of the literature on the interpretation of pain in the patient-physician encounter found that men reporting chronic pain were labeled "brave" by their practitioners, while women were labeled "emotional." Doctors were also more likely to initially conclude that women's pain was a signal of a mental rather than physical health condition.[27] A 2018 survey by members of the Department of Clinical Health Psychology at the University of Florida found that even female physicians and dentists described female patients as overreporting their pain.[28] What are the consequences for these biased interpretations of pain reports?

When physicians systematically do not acknowledge the symptom complaints of a category of patients, the consequence can be delayed diagnoses. A comprehensive population-wide analysis of disease progression patterns in Denmark found that across hundreds of diseases, women waited an average of four more years for a final diagnosis than did their male counterparts. For cancer, the average was 2.5 additional years. For metabolic diseases, such as diabetes, it was 4.5 years.[29,30] And even once a diagnosis is confirmed, differential interpretations of symptom discomfort based on the sex of the patient can result in inadequate symptom management and deepening distrust in the healthcare system.[31]

Social scientists need to develop new agendas to better study the impacts of ethnicity, race, and sex in the treatment of pain in particular and more generally in the experience of healthcare. The biased treatment of patients—not based on objective assessments of biological markers but based on the disparity in the interpretation of patients' narratives—can result in the dangerous and potentially deadly avoidance of medical care.[32]

My Brief Dance with Denial

I knew these facts when I felt that pain in my arm and shoulder. So, why did I often try to dismiss my own pain and symptoms? Beyond the structural and cultural factors that keep someone from seeking medical care, getting sick goes against the story we take pride in telling ourselves on an individual level.

In the beginning of my own experience, I could not face the fact that something could be seriously wrong. The disconnect between my pre-cancer life and the moment the orthopedist told me that the MRI results indicated the presence of cancer was not easily reconcilable. Before that first MRI, I was playing soccer once a week and squash twice a week before the shoulder and arm pain made that impossible. I was commuting to work, teaching all my classes, working in my garden, folding laundry, and shopping. Even after the first MRI, I continued to play soccer (I determined that I had better keep in shape in case I was facing a cancer diagnosis)—the orthopedic oncologist I saw right before my final diagnosis was a bit appalled at this news since I could have easily fractured my humerus during a fall.

As symptoms grow increasingly problematic, as the list of the normal activities in which we can participate increasingly diminishes, we seek a legitimate explanation for our suffering, for our inability to fulfill our duties. In my case, as the weeks and months progressed without a firm diagnosis—as each most likely cancer (breast, lung, colon) was ruled out and I continued to hold some hope that nothing was wrong—the progression of the disease and the accompanying pain screamed for my attention and demanded that I keep testing. I was transitioning into the sick role, despite my best efforts to avoid it.

In the previous chapter, I described sleeping upright, taking painkillers around the clock. Within a few weeks of that first emergency room visit, I could no longer use my right arm to drive, keeping it cradled on my lap as I commuted to work. I used my left arm to work the mouse on my computer, to wash my hair, to write on the board when I lectured. With each new limitation, as the burden of the illness and dysfunction grows, denial and avoidance transition into a desire to legitimate the experience—to embrace the sick role—to hopefully identify effective ways to resume function. I transitioned from wanting to run away from a serious diagnosis to running headlong into the arms of a medical institution and medical team who could provide treatment and care.

Why Me?

As I came to grips with the reality of my illness, I experienced another frustration common to those in my position.

Humans long for certainty and control over their destinies. We want to be confident that the seeds we plant will produce the fruit we need to survive, that the shelters we build will last and protect us from the elements, that any investment of time, emotion, or money will pay off. We like rational expectations, the identification of cause-and-effect relationships. And yet we also understand that despite our very best efforts, there will always be factors beyond our control. The heavy rains will fall and crops will flood; hurricanes and earthquakes will destroy our fragile shelters; stock markets will rise and fall.

When faced with an illness experience, we seek to provide context for the cause, especially if the timing is disruptive. Trying to identify the cause has multiple purposes. It can help identify factors we might be able to control in the future to avoid a recurrence, and it provides us an opportunity to "yell at the universe," to express our frustration at having our efforts and desires thwarted and for our bad luck.

A head cold that at any time might be annoying might be more upsetting for the college student during final exams or for the athlete competing in an important competition. (*I cannot believe I got sick right before final exams! I should have slept more. I should have taken better care of myself. Next time, I will know better. Why did this happen to me?*) We raise our eyes to the sky and ask, "Why me? Why now?" The more serious and, therefore, more disruptive the experience, the more poignant the question becomes. The "Why me?" question can be almost humorous for an untimely acute case of illness, allowing us to acknowledge the at-times absurdity of life, but it becomes graver after the diagnosis of chronic and/or life-threatening conditions.

Throughout history, some of the most common answers to the "Why me?" question in human communities have been to view illness as a curse or a punishment for some sin, even when the explanations combined biological and behavioral components. In the late seventeenth and eighteenth centuries, doctors attributed gout and syphilis to the loosening morals of the upper classes.[33] In the nineteenth century, patients' experience with tuberculosis was thought to help "purify" them.[33] Acknowledging this long history of the interpretation of illness as a result of sin remains a part of modern pastoral care, and it remains a core aspect of what Mike Bury refers to as the "core narratives" patients compose that reveal the meaning they give to their illness and suffering.[34,35]

But this answer does not serve all, as humans also struggle to understand why bad events happen to good people, a question memorably explored in Harold S. Kushner's 2004 book, *When Bad Things Happen to Good People.*[36] We also have daily examples of bad things *not* happening to bad people, the sinner *not* being punished. We only need to look at the front page of any newspaper around the world to witness accounts of corrupt and evil people wielding great power over good people and no "smiting" happening. The human experience is defined by an at-times incomprehensible combination of logic, intention, and chaos.

Years before my own cancer experience, I explored how cancer patients grappled with the "Why me?" question. When I was in college, in 1985, I spent one summer working as an intern for a start-up company producing continuing medical education videotapes. The particular tape we produced was designed to help pediatricians diagnose children with brain tumors. It was a fascinating opportunity that led to me to volunteer for a number of years at the Ronald McDonald House in Philadelphia and to write my master's thesis in 1991 on how families who had children survive pediatric cancer created narratives that helped them make sense of and gain some control over their experiences.[37] One of the key challenges faced by the families in my study was identifying the cause of their child's cancer. For many of these families, the cancer was diagnosed so early in the child's life that the oncologists assured the parents that "nothing they had done," no lifestyle choices or behaviors, no toxic exposure to carcinogens, had caused their child's cancer. It was simply a matter of "bad luck." While we might suspect that this information would be a source of solace for the families, it was not.

The families I interviewed did not attribute their child's cancer to sin, not their own and surely not their child's. In most of these cases, the child was so young when diagnosed, it would be hard to conceive of any sin they could have committed that would be so grave as to be punishable by a life-threatening cancer. But instead of providing comfort, being told by the medical team that "nothing you did caused your child's cancer" produced an uncertainty that challenged these parents in two fundamental ways—it challenged their role as parents, and it challenged their ability to return home after treatment.

A core parenting duty is to protect your children until they can take care of themselves. Parents feed, dress, bathe, and shelter their children, protecting them from hunger, exposure, and disease. They teach them about dangers in their environment. *(Don't touch the electrical socket! Always looks both ways before crossing the street!)* But how does a parent protect their child from a random, unlucky cellular malfunction? And if you cannot protect them, how do you manage that uncertainty? How do you continue to parent when faced with the brutal realization that you had no control over your child developing a life-threatening condition?

In response to these devastating questions, the parents in my study created origin stories—they developed their own answers to the "Why my child?" question. They focused on potential causes of their children's cancer, combining and employing facts they knew about known carcinogens and identifying the moment or moments their children were exposed, even though they understood that their oncologists would never validate these narratives as reasonable explanations (and, therefore, they never shared these narratives with their doctors). Their narratives incorporated recognizable causative elements—such as exposure to carcinogens—but lacked testable evidence or failed to demonstrate the necessary prolonged exposure necessary to claim a cause-and-effect event, a type of narrative Bury describes as "contingent narratives."[36] In their narratives, parents' decisions were often the source of the exposure event—a bad decision or some bad practices led to the child being exposed, often while in utero. But their actions were not sinful but rather the terrible cost of the infinite decisions we make every day, trying to fulfill our social obligations. For one family, the carcinogens the father brought home on his work clothes after working shifts at a wood treatment plant triggered their child's cancer. For one mother, it was a now-regrettable drive near the Three Mile Island nuclear plant when she was pregnant—not on the day of the accident at the plant in 1979 but before the cleanup of the site was finished in 1991.[38] For another mother, it was driving through northern New Jersey, near the gas refineries and the Newark Airport, while she was pregnant, an area that remains cited for some of the worst air pollution in the nation.[39]

The father had to keep working to support his family. The two mothers were fulfilling other competing family obligations. They were doing their best.

We might assume that accepting this narrative of responsibility would result in deep guilt, and yes, these parents did feel guilty about what they in hindsight defined as unfortunate decisions, but they also felt empowered. In acknowledging the mistakes, they gained insight into why their children's cancer had occurred, and now that they knew why, they felt empowered to *prevent* another exposure. "Now, we can protect our children," they thought. "Now, we can be good parents."

The imagined ability to identify the substance that caused their child's cancer provided the parents with a plan to resume their protective role. They identified a way to be a better parent, to not repeat a mistake. For many of these families, it also provided a way to return home. If the exposure had been identified as being near or around the home, parents proactively worked to clean or alter the home environment to reduce or remove the suspected carcinogen. This ritual was very important, as none of the families had the financial or emotional means to move to a "safer" neighborhood once the children were released from treatment.

We know from numerous studies of a multitude of patients with various serious conditions that patients will confront this "Why?" question at some time during their illness experience. And we know that the question has no clear answer. Many patients will conjure an answer that makes sense to them, that fits within their life narratives, or they will manage to live with the uncertainty, make peace with the concept of random bad luck and forces outside their control.

As we learn more about the human body and the ultimate causes of disease, even for the rare pediatric cancer, can we assume that the "Why me?" question will eventually have a clear medical explanation? And will the scientific answer then suffice? In short, no, because ultimately, the question we ask in the face of illness, and especially serious illness, is not about biological pathways and causative agents; it is about the meaning of one's life from the most personal, intimate perspective. Think of cases in which the physician might even be able to identify the causative agent. Think of the lifetime heavy smoker who gets diagnosed with lung cancer. Why me, Doctor? Well, we know that there is a correlation between smoking and the likelihood of developing lung cancer, so, why you? Because you have been a heavy smoker all your life. But this response does not answer the patient's question. Yes, smoking increases the risk of developing lung cancer, but only 24.4% of male heavy smokers and 18.5% of female heavy smokers will develop lung cancer.[40] So, why me? Well, it likely has to do with your genes, making you more susceptible to the destructive impacts of smoking. But why my genes, Doctor? Why did I end up with that particular genetic composition? Ultimately, no medical answer will fully satisfy.

Since the biological answer will fall short, like our forebears, we might conclude that our misfortune is the result of the ill-will of others, a curse. Others will continue to employ religious frameworks that argue that their illness is part of their gods' difficult-to-understand plan for them; even though that plan is beyond their comprehension because they are only human, it is okay, because the illness and suffering have ultimate meaning. And our answers can change as we learn more about the disease, as we interpret our journey through treatment, and as we hopefully prepare for our post-illness lives.

Why Me? My Personal Response

Like the families I studied, I was told by my oncologist and orthopedic oncologist that nothing I had done caused me to develop lymphoma; it was just "bad luck." From what the medical community understands about lymphoma, it does not arise from poor lifestyle choices.

Based on my family history, I knew what my health risks were likely to be as I got older and what conditions I could possibly avoid or minimize by making certain proactive lifestyle choices. My mother developed type 2 diabetes in her forties, and then in her early sixties, she developed colon and fallopian cancer (dying from a recurrence of the fallopian cancer at sixty-five). My father developed high blood pressure in his teens and died of a massive heart attack at sixty-nine. In response to their experiences, I adopted behaviors to reduce these particular risks. I eat a very high-fiber diet. I exercise multiple times a week. I drink plenty of water. I get regular screenings (I'm stretching the truth here a bit—I'm not always good with the screenings, especially GYN screenings). I tracked my blood pressure very closely over the years, and when it seemed to be creeping up a few years ago, I asked my primary care physician to prescribe blood pressure meds. And all the tests and scans that I had in search of the lymphoma suggested that these lifestyle choices are working to reduce my risk of developing the chronic diseases I seem genetically predestined to experience. None of my blood tests ever noted high blood sugar. My mammogram and CAT scans showed that my reproductive organs looked great. My colonoscopy was clear. My blood pressure is now well-controlled with low-dose lisinopril, and the ultrasound of my heart showed a healthy ticker. Being told that "nothing I did" caused me to develop lymphoma was simultaneously oddly comforting and very disconcerting. I was brutally reminded, as so many of us are, that I am not necessarily the master of my destiny, and while in our modern culture, we are made to feel so responsible for our own health, we are *not* fully responsible.[41,42] While we can proactively make some healthy choices, our individual health—and the health of the wider population—lies in the hands of structural, cultural, and environmental forces beyond any individual's control.

As modernizing societies have increasingly relied on the development and use of heavy metals and synthetic chemicals to fuel our industries and make our goods, and with the subsequent release of said chemicals into the environment as a result of production or use, physicians and epidemiologists have been tracking and testing how the human body processes these chemicals. In a 1968 article, Henry A. Schroeder and Isabel H. Tipton note the abundant presence of lead in human bodies living near highways and attribute this burden of lead, a toxic substance, to airborne lead from car exhaust.[43] (At the time, lead was being added to gasoline as an anti-knocking agent.) In 1987, Cancer Alley, an eighty-five-mile stretch of land housing more than 150 petrochemical plants in Louisiana between Baton Rouge and New Orleans, got its name after local residents raised the alarm about the unusually high rate of cancer cases in their communities, a finding confirmed by epidemiologists.[44] Studies have found that even the most health-conscious people have carcinogens and other harmful chemicals in their bodies, the result of our use of plastics (especially in regards to food packaging and storage), cosmetics, and cleaning products and from all the chemicals in the air and water that we breathe and drink every day. Medical scientists tracking the accumulated impact of these chemicals on our health refer to their presence as our "body burden," and the growing interest in their effects has led to the development of the field of exposomics.[45] The field has a lot of work to do. Of the tens of thousands of commercial chemicals we use, scientists have studied the health impacts of only roughly fifty to one hundred.[46] While we know the health risks and impacts associated with some individual chemicals, we know very little about the interactions of multiple chemicals in the body. Given how embedded these chemicals are in every aspect of our modern lives—our food, our hygiene products, our technology, our fuels—they cannot be completely avoided, even by the most informed, most proactive consumer. Individuals are limited—greater regulation would require government action to reduce our regular exposure to these substances. We humans are social animals living in a society whose environment places us at risk of exposure to dangerous substances and to the viruses among us. We all get sick, despite our best efforts.

Even though I recognize the limits of my agency and my responsibility, at the diagnostic stage of my experience, I found myself occasionally sulking and wishing that I had had a better return on all the health investments I had made already. I desperately wanted to go back a few weeks, a few months, and dodge this particular bullet. I wanted a benign explanation for the original odd MRI results of the scan of my humerus. I wanted to get a call from a medical professional telling me, "We're so sorry. The machine was not calibrated correctly! We made a mistake." But that call never came.

What answer did I provide when I wrestled with the "Why me?" question? After many fatigue-induced tears and heavy sighs, I was content sitting with the "bad luck" scenario, being the social scientist that I am. When I think for a minute about the countless biochemical actions that my body successfully completes every single day, it is actually amazing that so much goes right so much of the time! But I also know that many people struggle with probabilistic thinking, and sitting where I am would be distressing for them. As a sociologist who teaches research methods and quantitative analysis, I regularly read articles about how hard some students find the concept of probability, as it helps with my course development. These articles have helped me understand why teaching basic statistics can be so challenging. Even though children explore the concept of probability in many games they play growing up, where success might depend on the desired outcome of the roll of the dice, I marvel at how many actions we take, even while playing those childhood games, to attempt to influence the outcome. We blow on the dice! We shake them in our hands four times! We wear our lucky socks every time we play the game! When confronting random outcomes, we humans will try many different means to try to convince the universe to treat us well, to provide the lucky roll we need right now. So, while my lymphoma was just rotten bad luck, a case of cellular division gone awry, I, like many other patients, planned small rituals to help ensure that the outcome of my efforts to get better might work, to address and hopefully reduce the lingering uncertainty between my diagnosis and prognosis.[47] For every inpatient infusion, I would wear my new lucky socks (pink and gray stripes, with rubber bumps on the soles to prevent slipping). Hear my pleas, universe.

I also recognized that I could take some real actions to increase the chances that my treatment would work. My medical team encouraged me to get as much exercise as I could tolerate, try to stay as healthy as possible, and drink plenty of water, especially during and after chemotherapy treatments, actions I could take to maintain some sense of control beyond sock rituals! But even with my understanding and acceptance of random events, there were times throughout my cancer experience when an overwhelming shroud of despair at my powerlessness overwhelmed me, leaving me temporarily immobile, shaking my head and fighting back tears. My ritualistic response in this case? Get up, take my dogs for as long a walk as I could, drink a large glass of water, and breathe, often and deeply.

Interpreting the Prognosis

After trying to comprehend an often-devastating cancer diagnosis, during the first visit with the oncologist(s), patients grapple with trying to understand the requirements of treatments and, perhaps even more importantly, the prognosis. The copious details of treatment can wash over the patient like a turbulent wave as the oncologist or members of the medical team share an often-hurried yet complicated description of what chemotherapeutic or immunological materials they are likely to receive, what other treatments might be necessary (surgery, perhaps, or radiation), and the timing and duration of treatment(s). Patients may feel as though they are drowning in all of this information. Medical personnel supplement the verbal descriptions with a folder or binder for the patient, replete with documents that can be reviewed at a later time. The medical staff member reviewing the information admits, "I know that this is a lot of information to hear right now," and yet there can be no delay in sharing it, no stepwise review of material today, with the rest to be covered tomorrow or the next day. The cancer diagnosis requires a quick and aggressive response by the oncology team. Delaying treatment any longer than it was already delayed before the illness was diagnosed can threaten successful treatment. While the urgency to intervene as soon as possible makes medical sense, trying to comprehend all the details, often presented in a specialized language foreign to those without medical training and, therefore, written at literacy levels higher than those of the average American patient, makes a patient's attempt to be informed about what will happen next extremely challenging.[48,49,50] The patient may have neither the vocabulary nor the calm rational bandwidth needed to comprehend what they are hearing or reading. It often takes time before a patient can even start coming close to grasping all the changes that are about to happen.

A cancer prognosis is often described in terms of the percentage of people who achieve remission—that is, the state at which no active cancer can be detected. Remission statistics reflect trends for the general population, not for individuals. Often presented in technical statistical and mathematical references—rates, risks, ratios—they can be confusing for individuals to interpret.[51,52] Due to often-significant risks of recurrence for many cancers, oncologists typically do not talk about cure rates until a patient has remained cancer-free for anywhere between five and ten years. The range of five-year remission rates varies considerably based on the type of cancer, from a low of less than 1% for patients with cancer of the brain stem to a high of 98% for patients diagnosed with prostate cancer.[53] But how do patients interpret these percentages? As noted earlier, people struggle with probabilistic thinking.

From patients I have interviewed during my graduate training in the 1990s and more recently, and while interacting with patients during my own cancer experience, I learned that they are often acutely aware that although the remission rate is, say, 80%, their personal experience will be either 0% or 100%. Most patients are very aware that they will either survive this illness episode, or they will not. They know that they will not get 80% better.

Given this understanding, patients will often try to get clues from the medical team about which category they might fall into or try to figure out how to maximize their chance of getting into the survivor's category. Many of the families with whom I interacted who experienced pediatric cancer reported often being surprised about who did and did not survive among the children with this diagnosis. They noted, for example, the lack of expected correlation between tolerance of the surgery, chemotherapy, or radiation and survival. Sometimes, the "strongest" (those who seemed to tolerate treatments well) passed, while the "weakest" (those who had severe side effects) survived. While this correlation may not make sense if we assume that the "strong" will have the greatest chance of survival, the opposite might counterintuitively be the better predictor. If the degree of side effects a patient experiences signals that the treatment is indeed killing cells—cancerous and, unfortunately in the short term, healthy cells—then the "weak" might be displaying a greater and, therefore, better response to treatment. Some studies of certain cancers demonstrate this correlation—the greater the side effects from the current treatment protocols, the better the chance of survival.[54,55]

Patients and family members talk about their frustration over their physicians not telling them whether they think that they or their sick family member will "make it," even when directly asked.[56] It makes sense why a physician would not share their own experiential-based "gut" feelings with a patient about their likelihood of survival, even though we all suspect, as they are sitting there across from us, reviewing our charts and taking our vitals, that they have a sense about which of us will survive. But their reticence serves themselves and their patients. Our physicians need to start off the process fully engaged and committed to the patient before them. They have to have hope to maintain that investment. They also need to give us hope, as we will be asked to allow the poisons to flow through our veins if we have any chance for survival. They also hesitate because from their experience, they know that their gut feelings are not always right. They have also been surprised by who did or did not successfully complete treatment. And as Renée C. Fox richly describes in her classic study, *Experiment Perilous*, in the face of uncertainly, even our highly rational and scientific physicians will engage in lucky rituals, casting hopeful "bets" in their attempts to help their patients.[57] But during our appointments, we patients still try to get them to show "specific optimism" toward our case, not just "general optimism." The positive statements they do share—"Your blood counts look great today! You seem to be tolerating everything very well! You seem to have good healing ability!"—ring much louder in our ears, and our step is a bit lighter as we walk out of the exam room. Patients and the people supporting them focus more directly on and hear a bit more clearly any suggestion of good news.[58]

But even though we might know that we cannot and should not try to pin our medical practitioners down, we often cannot help ourselves. I tried this tactic on my orthopedic oncologist when I went in for a consultation for my bone biopsy. I pushed her on whether she thought, from the limited information she had, that I ultimately would be "okay," and she kindly but firmly told me that she really could not say until they did the biopsy and she could "see" the cells. I do recall, however, that she said, "If we have to find something, we hope it is lymphoma, because we have a lot of tools at our disposal for lymphoma." Perhaps I did get her to share her own gut feeling or hopeful ritual in the end? I was told by my oncologist at my first appointment that the current remission rate for my type of lymphoma in response to the treatment protocol, R-CHOP, is 70%. And my thoughts immediately turned to "Okay, but what are *my* chances?"

Factors That Help Us Survive

From the analysis of large data sets, oncologists know that many biological factors are associated with a greater chance of surviving all cancers combined, including age, general state of overall health, the stage and spread of the cancer, and specific factors of the cancer cells themselves (for example, degree of chromosomal abnormalities). But social and structural factors can also help individuals fall into the survivors category. I am very aware of all the "factors in my favor" since I occupy many of the favorable categories. My recognition of the powerful impacts of these social determinants of health has long informed my advocating for universal healthcare throughout my professional career.

Higher Education and Employment

People with higher education tend to have better survival outcomes. It is not hard to identify some of the causal mechanisms here; people with higher education tend to have better employment opportunities, which often translate into work with flexibility, autonomy, security, health insurance, and higher incomes. Higher education also facilitates communication with medical practitioners and the ability to advocate for your needs in medical settings.

As a college professor, I was extremely fortunate to have an employer that worked with me so that I could take a leave of absence during my treatment. In hindsight, I could not imagine how I would have managed teaching, given the extreme fatigue I experienced as a result of treatment. My colleagues picked up the extra work my unexpected leave created, and they never made me feel guilty.

I could not imagine having to go directly from a chemotherapy infusion to my workplace, and yet I saw this happen firsthand. Plenty of patients I saw each time I went into Philadelphia for my infusions did not have the luxury of going home to recuperate after a procedure; they had to keep working to keep their health insurance and bring home an income. While for some, continuing to work provides some normalcy during the medical crisis, for others, it is an overwhelming burden.[59]

Recent studies have shown that a cancer diagnosis significantly increases the chance of job loss, a risk faced by the 45% of people diagnosed with cancer in the United States who fall within the traditional working-age cohort of twenty to sixty-four.[60] While the risk of job loss varies by the type of cancer and the demands of treatment (including length of treatment and side effects' impact on ability to function), patients with manual labor jobs, those with lower-income jobs, those with jobs with lower educational requirements, and females face the greatest risk of losing employment, especially since these workers are often working at businesses exempt from having to provide employment protections guaranteed by the Americans with Disabilities Act and the Family and Medical Leave Act.[61] And only about 54% of working-age cancer survivors work full-time after treatment.[62] Patients who lose their income or face significant financial burdens, including bankruptcy, during or after treatment have double the mortality rate.[63] In the United States, 62% of patients go into debt due to their treatments, 55% accrue at least $10,000 in debt, 42% report losing their life savings, and 3% file for bankruptcy.[64,65]

"Good" Health Insurance

Cancer patients with health insurance have significantly better treatment outcomes than the uninsured, in part because they receive a diagnosis and treatment at earlier stages in their disease state. But there are also gradients by type of insurance, with private insurance plans and Medicare often outperforming Medicaid and other public programs in providing timely and comprehensive care and buffering against unmanageable out-of-pocket costs.[66] The particular health insurance coverage provided by my employer provided me access to one of the top cancer treatment centers in the world, Penn Medicine's Abramson Cancer Center in Philadelphia. I had no doubt from the very start of my experience that I would be receiving the best cancer care anyone in the United States could hope to access. My coverage was comprehensive, so I was able to manage the minimal out-of-pocket expenses that I incurred.

Shelter, Nutrition, and Sanitation

The human organism needs three basic provisions to live—adequate shelter, sufficient nutrition (including food and water), and adequate sanitation. If any of these are insufficient, an individual may not thrive or survive. They remain important basic components of human health throughout our lives   people who have lost their homes or live in poor housing, whose diets are deficient, and who cannot maintain their hygiene experience higher rates of morbidity and mortality.[67,68,69,70]

The quality of one's shelter during cancer treatment is important not only as a basic component of general health but as a way to minimize the risk of secondary infections during treatment. Many cancer treatment protocols render the patient at least temporarily immunocompromised. At the time of my diagnosis and during treatment, I lived in a house in a suburb of Philadelphia with my husband and my two dogs. Our two children were old enough to be living independently. It was very easy to control my exposure to people when I was immunocompromised, especially since I was able to take time off from work. My husband was diligent about his exposure to anyone who might be contagious in his work setting, and we had a ritual of washing or sanitizing our hands whenever we came into the house. Living with a supportive partner meant that I had someone who could run errands, do laundry, and take the dogs for a walk whenever the side effects from treatment impaired me. My house has functioning air-conditioning, so although many of my treatments happened during the summer months, I could keep cool and sleep comfortably. I could take a bath or shower whenever I wanted. In a house equipped with a washer and dryer, I could launder my clothes and bedding as often as needed. My dishwasher could sanitize my dishes. And as I acknowledged the importance of each of these basic assets I had, my thoughts turned to the patient living in a crowded apartment with no washer and dryer, no dishwasher, no air-conditioning.

Another factor that promotes treatment success is a heart-healthy diet, with a focus on good proteins. Given that nausea and constipation are typical side effects from treatment, eating well can be an incredible challenge. And yet given the cellular destruction from treatment, the body's nutritional demands are high. As noted earlier, even before my cancer diagnosis, I enjoyed preparing and eating a healthy diet, and for the most part, I continued to enjoy that diet throughout treatment. I am very fortunate to have access to fresh, healthy foods within walking distance of my house, so even on my worst days, I could still access and pay for nutritional foods. In 2013, about 14.3% of Americans were food-insecure. A recent study of cancer patients in New Mexico found that 26% of a sample of patients with breast, colorectal, or prostate cancer reported being food-insecure at the time of diagnosis and during treatment. But 10% of these patients experienced food insecurity *after* their diagnosis, in part as a result of the new financial burdens associated with treatment.[71] Medical practitioners and investigators interested in addressing disparities in cancer care are calling for more research into the phenomenon of cancer diagnoses causing food insecurity.[72,73]

Exercise

An increasing number of studies have shown a positive link between exercising during cancer treatment and surviving cancer. Patients who exercise have a lower risk of mortality and recurrence and better manage their treatment's side effects. As such, exercise is becoming a standard component of cancer care.[74] The motivation to exercise might be almost nonexistent when managing the most severe side effects of treatment, but care teams will keep encouraging patients to get as much as they can tolerate as often as possible.

Here, too, my social position gives me advantages that not all cancer patients enjoy. Living in a walkable suburb, I can exercise in my neighborhood at any time of the day or night and not worry about my safety. I have level, uncrowded sidewalks, a local college campus, and local nature preserves where I can get a daily dose of vigorous walking. I suspended my membership at a local health club since no matter how clean the facility is, these settings are not ideal for the immunocompromised. Plus, I primarily went to the club to play squash, and that would not be happening for a while once I started treatment. But a limited percentage of Americans live in neighborhoods that are deemed walkable. A 2015 study found that only about 14% of all neighborhoods in metropolitan areas in the United States have good walkable access, yet 80% of Americans live in urban areas.[75] And beyond cancer survivorship, living in walkable, safe neighborhoods provides a number of general health benefits; as such, there are continued calls to developers for more concerted design efforts to make urban, suburban, and rural areas as walkable as possible.

It was unnervingly sobering and encouraging to recognize all of my advantages as I began my illness experience. I felt comforted that I could use all of my resources to hopefully survive this diagnosis, but the review of all of these barriers to health once again illuminated all the work needed to advocate for and secure better healthcare access for everyone.

About a week after my first outpatient chemotherapy infusion, my right arm felt much better. My mobility had not improved, but the pain was greatly reduced. I had no idea at that point whether the reduction in pain was an indication that the chemotherapy had started attacking the cancer cells or whether I was feeling relief from the post-chemo steroids, but I was anxious to interpret the relief as a much-needed sign of hope. Seeking signs of hope and taking whatever proactive measures I could would define my attempts to exert some control over my treatment experience.

The First Outpatient Infusions

Worse Than the Disease

As I shared in Chapter 2, my first treatments did bring some relief from the unbearable pain I was experiencing while waiting for my diagnosis. But as many cancer patients experience, my treatments also brought numerous debilitating and challenging side effects. For cancer patients, these side effects may add to the impairments they were experiencing prior to diagnosis, making the treatment experience feel "worse than the disease." The side effects might also be worse than the original presenting symptoms of cancer at the time of diagnosis.

The list of common symptoms of cancer are numerous and often vague. As noted in the previous chapter, until symptoms impede our ability to fulfill our normative roles, it is tempting to ignore them as indications of benign and/or acute maladies. Most of us do not go willingly into the sick role. Even the American Cancer Society notes that any of the following common symptoms of cancer might be caused by another problem:

- Fatigue or extreme tiredness that doesn't get better with rest.
- Weight loss or gain of ten pounds or more for no known reason
- Eating problems such as not feeling hungry, trouble swallowing, belly pain, or nausea and vomiting
- Swelling or lumps anywhere in the body
- Thickening or lump in the breast or other part of the body

- Pain, especially new or with no known reason, that doesn't go away or gets worse
- Skin changes such as a lump that bleeds or turns scaly, a new mole or a change in a mole, a sore that does not heal, or a yellowish color to the skin or eyes (jaundice)
- Cough or hoarseness that does not go away
- Unusual bleeding or bruising for no known reason
- Change in bowel habits, such as constipation or diarrhea, that doesn't go away or a change in how your stools look
- Bladder changes such as pain when passing urine, blood in the urine, or needing to pass urine more or less often
- Fever or nights sweats
- Headaches
- Vision or hearing problems
- Mouth changes such as sores, bleeding, pain, or numbness[1]

At the beginning stages of disease progression, many of these symptoms may be minor enough not to impede with the fulfillment of normative roles, even if they are deemed annoying. They might also be explained by recent activity, stress and anxiety, an injury, allergies, or a possible foodborne illness. And it is difficult for patients to assess how long the symptoms need to be experienced before they can no longer be explained by recent events and require attention.

According to recommendations on the National Cancer Institute's (NCI's) website, experiencing any of these aforementioned symptoms for more than "a few weeks" is a cause for concern.[2] But even the NCI's use here of the qualifier *few* (as compared to the phrase *a couple of*) complicates interpretation, as *few* is used in contrast to *many*, but both terms are scalable.[3] Compare my meaning when I refer to the few stars I can see in the sky at night compared to the many that I know exist versus the few days every month that I make time to work on a beloved hobby. In both descriptions, the listener can interpret my meaning, but no definite number is applied. *Few* in the first example refers to the "small" number I can see (perhaps about seventy in my suburban night sky that are visible with the naked eye) compared to the approximately ten thousand (again, visible with the naked eye) that exist.[4] In the second example, *few* would likely suggest a small number (perhaps between three and seven) compared to the roughly thirty days in a month.

Research also shows that our ability to accurately recall how long we have experienced symptoms is greatly impaired by a variety of factors, including our emotional states, levels of anxiety, the persistent or intermittent experience of the symptom(s), and whether the symptom(s) coincide with other "landmarking" events in our lives, such as holidays or other momentous transitions.[5,6] Understandable ignoring or downplaying of symptoms may contribute to delayed diagnoses. Recall that any discomfort I felt in my shoulder prior to the night I ended up in the emergency room could have been attributed to a sports activity.

Unlike my experience, about 50% or more of cancer patients do not experience pain as one of the main symptoms. Many cancer patients were relatively healthy before their cancer diagnosis.[7] Relative underlying good health, the absence of pain, and the minimal impact of some symptoms are contributing factors to why some cancer patients experience treatment as being worse than the disease. The challenge medical practitioners face is convincing patients that they must feel worse to hopefully get the cancer in remission. And a challenge for the patient is to interpret the side effects as evidence that they are doing what they need to do—they are fulfilling one of their sick-role obligations.

Nonmaleficence

Since cancer treatments kill cancerous and healthy cells, causing some damage to healthy tissue, they violate one of the core principles of bioethics medical professionals follow to inform their care decisions: nonmaleficence. The four core principles are autonomy, nonmaleficence, beneficence, and justice.[8] Thomas McCormick from the University of Washington School of Medicine provides these succinct definitions of the principles:

1. Respect for Autonomy

Any notion of moral decision-making assumes that rational agents are involved in making informed and voluntary decisions. In health care decisions, our respect for the autonomy of the patient would, in common parlance, imply that the patient has the capacity to act intentionally, with understanding, and without controlling influences that would mitigate against a free and voluntary act. This principle is the basis for the practice of "informed consent" in the physician/patient transaction regarding health care.

2. The Principle of Nonmaleficence

The principle of nonmaleficence requires of us that we not intentionally create a harm or injury to the patient, either through acts of commission or omission. In common language, we consider it negligent if one imposes a careless or unreasonable risk of harm upon another. Providing a proper standard of care that avoids or minimizes the risk of harm is supported not only by our commonly held moral convictions, but by the laws of society as well. This principle affirms the need for medical competence. It is clear that medical mistakes may occur; however, this principle articulates a fundamental commitment on the part of health care professionals to protect their patients from harm.

3. The Principle of Beneficence
The ordinary meaning of this principle is that health care providers have a duty to be of a benefit to the patient, as well as to take positive steps to prevent and to remove harm from the patient. These duties are viewed as rational and self-evident and are widely accepted as the proper goals of medicine. This principle is at the very heart of health care implying that a suffering supplicant (the patient) can enter into a relationship with one whom society has licensed as competent to provide medical care, trusting that the physician's chief objective is to help. The goal of providing benefit can be applied both to individual patients, and to the good of society as a whole. For example, the good health of a particular patient is an appropriate goal of medicine, and the prevention of disease through research and the employment of vaccines is the same goal expanded to the population at large.

4. The Principle of Justice
Justice in health care is usually defined as a form of fairness, or as Aristotle once said, "giving to each that which is his due." This implies the fair distribution of goods in society and requires that we look at the role of entitlement. The question of distributive justice also seems to hinge on the fact that some goods and services are in short supply, there is not enough to go around, thus some fair means of allocating scarce resources must be determined.[9]

The principle of nonmaleficence is also often concisely summed by the moral imperative of "first, do no harm," a phrase attributed to Hippocrates.[10] There are many examples where medical treatments in general and cancer treatments in particular cause harm, so the lens through which we judge whether they are ethical cannot be solely on the basis of whether they cause *any* harm but rather on the basis of whether they are being administered in response to a patient's autonomous decision to undergo treatment and whether they are the patient's best chance for survival, thereby giving a greater priority to the principle of beneficence. The exorbitant cost of cancer treatments tragically results in our paying the least attention to the principle of justice.

But preparing patients for the very likely experience of extreme side effects from treatment is not an easy task for the oncology team. The oncologist often does not bring the patient immediate or quick relief from their symptoms and suffering but rather prescribes a treatment protocol that sends them deeper into suffering in the hopes that they might arise later, in remission and feeling better. This reality challenges our concepts of the relationship between physician and patient and our expected outcome of submitting to the power and authority of the medical professional. I am sick, suffering. I come to you, and you make me feel better by restoring me to my previous state of health or as close to that previous state as you can.

This challenge of accepting that you will have to feel worse before you can possibly feel better has a correlate in the realm of general fitness culture, and that is the concept of "no pain, no gain." This phrase became embedded in our common fitness vernacular as a result of its frequent use in Jane Fonda's fitness videos of the 1980s.[11] When we exercise hard, we force our muscles to work beyond the availability of the oxygen supply in our blood, therefore impeding complete cellular respiration and resulting in the formation of lactic acid. The formation of lactic acid forces more blood flow to the impacted muscles, resulting in greater future strength and endurance.[12] So, for some activities, "pain" can result in "gain." But a very small minority of cancer patients will come out of their cancer experience with greater strength and endurance at the end of treatment than they had before. And a phrase such as "no strife, no 'chance for' life" just does not have the same catchy ring.

Ways to Make It Less "Worse"?

Some medical professionals argue that trying to minimize the impact of the side effects may go a long way in minimizing the trauma of cancer treatments and may reduce the number of patients who refuse to start treatment or stop treatment as a result of the side effects. About 1% of patients refuse treatment, while studies suggest that about 3%–19% of patients refuse some component(s) of their treatment protocol.[13,14,15] Not surprisingly, having poor survival prospects increases the chance of not starting or stopping treatment—a potentially rational calculation of costs and benefits. Older patients are also more likely not to start or stop, again, as a result of assessing that the cost of undergoing treatments is unlikely to significantly increase their life expectancy.

But for the patients who do start treatment, more proactive management of side effects may mitigate the sense that the treatment is worse than the disease and therefore increase compliance with the treatment protocol.[16] But for patients and practitioners, making the management of the side effects a priority may seem trivial compared to the bigger picture of saving a life. Some of the common side effects from cancer treatments include:[17]

Anemia
Appetite loss
Bleeding and bruising
    (thrombocytopenia)
Constipation
Delirium
Diarrhea
Edema (swelling)
Fatigue
Fertility issues in boys and men
Fertility issues in girls and
    women
Flulike symptoms
Hair loss (alopecia)
Infection and neutropenia
Lymphedema
Memory or concentration
    problems
Mouth and throat problems
Nausea and vomiting
Nerve problems (peripheral
    neuropathy)
Organ-related inflammation and
    immunotherapy
Pain
Sexual health issues in men
Sexual health issues in women
Skin and nail changes
Sleep problems
Urinary and bladder problems

From the perspective of the patient and their medical team, treating these side effects is less dire and essential than stopping the spread of the cancer and hopefully destroying the cancer already present. Actually addressing the discomfort of these side effects, however, provides an opportunity for medical and other caregivers to acknowledge the patient's illness narrative, appreciating the details. The patient can be grateful that they have accessed treatment while still benefitting from a chance to grumble and receive some comfort. The patient can fully understand that the significant fatigue, the nausea and constipation, the odd changes to the skin are expected and unavoidable side effects of the chemotherapy, but brushing off these discomforts as insignificant complaints "in the big picture" misses the opportunity to hold the patient facing their own mortality connected to the social world. It misses an opportunity to provide relief from suffering, one of the expected results of the physician/medical team and patient interaction and the kinds of interactions that bind us to each other in wider society. A well-timed Zofran tablet,[18] a drug that blocks the actions of chemicals in the body that can trigger nausea and vomiting, might help address a patient's nausea, but a Zofran tablet given with a fresh glass of water by someone taking even a moment to acknowledge the challenge of feeling nauseated so often, provides the added needed balm for a struggling spirit.

I can remember clearly when my doctor told me that I would lose my hair, about two weeks after receiving the first outpatient infusion. For all the research I had done on cancer patients, for all the research I had done on my form of lymphoma prior to my first appointment with the oncologist, I had not realized that this reality would be mine, as even though hair loss is a common side effect, it is not everyone's experience. The news should not have surprised me, but it caught me completely off guard, and I started to cry. It was important at that moment that I be allowed to cry, even for just a minute or two, as this news harshly drove home the point that my illness experience was going to get worse before I could possibly get better. I kept asking myself, "How could I have missed this information? How could I have not realized?"

Most of the comforting and acknowledging of the side effects are delivered by the nursing staff in medical settings and by select family members and friends in other settings. Referring to the principles of bioethics, we can contemplate why physicians would find it hard to acknowledge the pain and suffering that their prescribed interventions cause. Oncologists must focus on the desired ultimate outcome of these aggressive and challenging treatments—getting their patients into remission. From countless conversations I have had with my own physicians and with those whom I have professionally studied, I know that they find it incredibly difficult to see their patients in pain. To see a patient suffering and to know that there are no guarantees that the suffering will be rewarded with survival highlights physicians' struggle to fulfill their ethical duty to maximize beneficence and minimize maleficence. Some studies have recorded discordance between physicians' and patients' assessment of the prevalence, duration, and severity of side effects, with physicians underestimating or inadequately responding to patients' concerns.[19,20] The task of providing comfort, since the cause of the suffering remains medically necessary, therefore likely falls to nonphysicians.

We Are Not Autonomous: Who Comes
to the Appointments?

During my first oncology appointment, my doctor provided an overview of what my test results revealed and reviewed plans for beginning treatment. My husband attended this appointment with me, as I was sure that I would need an extra set of ears to adequately hear even a fraction of the overwhelming amount of information we would cover. I also recognized that everything that I was going to directly face during treatment would also affect my husband. Beyond his emotional challenge of acknowledging the serious threat of possible death I was facing, we also understood that I would need his significant assistance to get to and from my medical appointments and that my side effects and possible impairments would affect the smooth operation of our shared household. We needed to hear the information together so that we could plan for how we might be able to minimize the disruption of our lives.

Studies show that having someone—a friend or caretaker—with you during medical appointments provides significant benefits, from supplying necessary emotional support to helping patients manage the flood of medical information. This benefit is especially true for patients facing serious medical conditions, who unquestionably need physical and emotional assistance, and for patients who might struggle to comprehend the diagnosis and treatment protocols (think of common vulnerable populations, such as children and people who are cognitively impaired). Having support during appointments increases the health literacy of the patient and the caretaker and increases the likelihood of positive outcomes.[21] A wealth of literature argues that care teams should pay more attention to the impact of a cancer diagnosis on a patient's formal and informal care networks since they both play a significant role in the patient's experience and outcome.[22]

While someone's accompanying a patient to an appointment has been shown to have benefits, their presence may also complicate the patient's exercise of autonomy. When someone other than the patient and the physician is in the room, can we be certain that the patient is exercising genuine autonomy in making decisions about their care? We often hope and trust that the accompanying person has a good relationship with the patient and wants them to get better, but given the financial and caretaking demands, might their presence potentially complicate the patient's and physician's informed-consent conversation? Might there be a temptation not to pursue some form of treatment precisely because the patient recognizes the types of financial, emotional, and/or physical burdens their decision might cause the family member(s) or friend in the room?

Bioethical debates in the United States often deem autonomy as the crowning principle.[23] American culture was built on an ideal of individualism derived from our Puritan roots. Early European migrants to America rejected the hierarchy of European monarchies and the hierarchy of the Catholic Church, seeking a new form of government—for and by the people, with representation—and a more direct relationship with the divine. In this new social experiment, the moral value of the individual was elevated and celebrated, with some positive outcomes, including increased chances for social mobility, ingenuity, specialization, and freedom of expression.

Focusing on the individual, however, also has some negative impacts. Concentrating on the individual inevitably draws attention away from our interconnectedness, both the degree to which we rely on others for their specialized labor and support and how as social creatures we crave social interaction. The emphasis on the individual also results in a form of social Darwinism,[24] where we attribute an individual's successes and failures to their own efforts—survival of the fittest—instead of recognizing how the structures and functions of social institutions and particular historical contexts influence our biographies beyond any of our personal initiatives and efforts.[25]

Being sick often reminds us, sometimes brutally, of our reliance on others and of the limits of our own efforts to avoid illness. The extent and duration of this reliance can be a significant challenge for the patient and their caregivers. While having others in the room when a patient is making decisions about their care by definition challenges the unfettered expression of the patient's autonomy, our lived reality outside the exam room demands that they be present. Who among us makes big life decisions, such as a move, job change, and so forth, without consulting all the people close to us who will be affected by those decisions?[26] Part of the genuine expression of our autonomy is, perhaps, counterintuitively making space to understand the patient's possibly complex or challenging support network and to recognize how the composition and characteristics of this particular network will affect the patient's experience. Providing this space and recognition has led to the development of the concept of "relational autonomy."[27,28,29]

Learning about New Drugs

My first outpatient infusion occurred on June 21, 2019. The appointment began with a blood test, followed by a quick appointment with my oncologist. Once my blood counts indicated that I was robust enough to get the infusion, I was sent to the infusion center down the hall. As soon as the pharmacy sent up my mix of chemicals—the right combination and correct dosage based on my weight—the infusion process began.

Before my first infusion, my care team shared handouts naming and describing all the drugs I would be receiving as part of my treatment protocol and their likely side effects. I was impressed that these materials were informative yet concise and written so they could be read by patients at varying degrees of education, even if the drug names and their scientific "classes" would not be familiar to the average patient. Currently, the average American reads at between a seventh- and eighth-grade level, so in the name of fulfilling the ethical obligation of obtaining informed consent in medical settings, all patient materials should be drafted accordingly. These materials are composed with the understanding that this level is an average and that about 21% of the general population has problems completing reading "tasks that require comparing and contrasting information, paraphrasing, or making low-level inferences."[30] No matter how carefully the materials are composed, some patients will need assistance with reading anything distributed by medical practitioners.

I often ask my students how many of them read the package inserts that come with their prescriptions. In a class of about thirty students, typically one student—about 3%—will raise their hand. This student tends to be majoring in the natural or health sciences. Why do so few of us read these inserts?

In 1966, the "Fair Packaging and Labeling Act required all consumer products in interstate commerce to be honestly and informatively labeled, with the FDA enforcing these provisions on foods, drugs, cosmetics, and medical devices."[31] In 2006, the law was expanded to more fully define the list of information that was required on prescription drugs' package inserts (see list on page 46). As Joseph P. Nathan and Etty Vider argue, the information in the packets is intended to be used by medical practitioners, not by the average patient. The inserts contain far more technical information than could be consumed by the average patient, are written at a level above the average literacy rate, and provide significantly more information than needed to meet the basic requirements of informed consent. The assumption is that the doctor or other allied health professional will educate a patient about a drug's use and risks. Legally, this assumption is termed the "learned intermediary doctrine."[32]

Contents of the Full Prescribing Information

The full prescribing information section of the package insert contains detailed information about the drug.[33] Specific information includes the following, in the order listed:

- Boxed warning
- Indications and usage
- Dosage and administration
- Dosage forms and strengths
- Contraindications
- Warnings and precautions
- Adverse reactions (specifically, adverse events for which there is some basis to believe that a causal relationship exists between the drug and the adverse event)
- Drug interactions (specifically, clinically significant interactions)
- Use in specific populations (pregnant women, nursing mothers, pediatrics, geriatrics, and other subpopulations)
- Drug abuse and dependence
- Overdosage
- Description (dosage form[s], ingredients, pharmacologic or therapeutic class, and other relevant information)
- Clinical pharmacology (mechanism of action, pharmacodynamics, and pharmacokinetics)
- Nonclinical toxicology (carcinogenesis, mutagenesis, impairment of fertility, and animal toxicology and/or pharmacology)
- Clinical studies
- References
- How it is supplied/storage and handling
- Patient counseling information

The problem is that this assumed exchange between patient and prescriber rarely occurs. While the prescriber often explains the rationale for writing a prescription, few, if any, then review in detail the risks or possible side effects with patients. We also rarely if ever fill and open our prescriptions in the presence of our prescribers. Our act of consent occurs when we hand the script to the pharmacist, accept and pay for the package, and then open and consume the drug according to the instructions. Few of us read the package insert for the commonly prescribed antibiotic, decongestant, or pain-relief medication because we trust that our physicians are trying to help and not harm us, we trust that any side effects will not be extreme, we already are aware that we are unlikely to understand the information on the insert, and we are likely not feeling good due to whatever ails us. All of these factors result in our tossing the insert unread into the garbage or recycling bin.

But when cancer patients are told from the start that the drugs we are about to take have potentially serious and life-altering side effects, despite trusting our doctors and believing that they want to help us, and while recognizing our own limited knowledge base, we might want to spend some time reviewing the handouts.

R-CHOP

My treatment protocol is called R-CHOP. It is a standard treatment protocol for diffuse large B cell lymphoma.

DRUGS IN THE R-CHOP COMBINATION

R= Rituximab
C= Cyclophosphamide
H= Doxorubicin hydrochloride (hydroxydaunomycin)
O= Vincristine sulfate (Oncovin)
P= Prednisone[34]

Rituximab is a monoclonal antibody that attaches itself to a specific protein found on the surface of healthy and cancerous B cells in our bodies. B cells are a normal component of our immune systems. Once the rituximab is attached, it sends instructions to the patient's immune system to destroy the cell. Patients are typically given an antihistamine before the infusion begins since allergic reactions can occur.

Cyclophosphamide is an alkylating agent that damages the DNA of cells, preventing them from dividing and causing them to die. Cells that divide quickly, such as cancer cells, are more sensitive to this process.

Doxorubicin hydrochloride is an anthracycline that, like cyclophosphamide, works at the level of DNA. It interrupts the copying of DNA, which
causes cancer cells to die. This particular drug is known colloquially as the
"Red Devil." It got this name in part because it is bright red, but the "devil"
tag is associated with the burning and/or painful sensation that patients often feel even when the drug is administered properly and there is no leakage
from the intravenous lines. It is also toxic to the heart—so toxic that every
individual has a lifetime maximum dosage that they can receive. Another
intriguing aspect of the drug is that it causes a patient's urine to temporarily
turn red while the body is circulating and processing the drug, a side effect
my nurses warned me about since patients not informed panic, thinking that
they are peeing blood!

Oncovin (vincristine) is a member of the vinca alkaloids family of drugs.
It works by interfering with cell division, impeding the cancer's ability to
grow and spread. My favorite fact about this drug is that it is derived from the
periwinkle plant. As I shared earlier, I love gardening, and this tidbit brought
me comfort as I read through my R-CHOP information sheets. This information made the drug I was going to receive seem natural and familiar, as I had
often planted periwinkle in my garden (it is sometimes called annual vinca
in gardening centers). A plant that I had cared for in my own garden space
was now going to take care of me and hopefully help me survive. Picturing a
blooming periwinkle helped me feel less afraid of the entire chemo cocktail.

Many readers will recognize that prednisone is a common, familiar steroid. It is taken with the infusion to help control post-exposure inflammation
and mitigate some of the side effects of the aforementioned drugs.

The First Outpatient Infusions

One lovely aspect of my first infusion was being able to have a private infusion room. This benefit was standard at the Perelman Center. Back in the late
1990s, I served as the support person during several of my mother's infusions
for fallopian cancer at the University of Pennsylvania, years before the con-
struction of the Perelman Center, and at that time, infusions occurred in a
spacious common room—no dividers. While a common room might provide
a sense of camaraderie, it does not allow for privacy.

My first room did not have a window, but it had a very comfortable reclining chair as well as an extra (not reclining and far less comfortable) chair for
a support person. I had gotten my "chemo port" implanted the day before. A

chemo port is a medical device that typically sits underneath your skin near the collarbone and facilitates access to a patient's veins.[35] The port itself is about the size of a quarter, with a central access site where medical staff can draw blood, administer drugs, or connect to an IV. A catheter tube extends off the center and connects directly to the jugular or subclavian vein. As soon as they accessed my port, I would be ready.

My port was apparently a very good port because throughout my outpatient and inpatient infusion experiences, the staff regularly complimented me on the port I had—a PowerPort by BD.[36] I laughed every time they complimented me since their praise suggested that I had made a "good choice." I wondered whether anyone thought that I had done research and consulted with *Consumer Reports* to make sure that I got the best one on the market. Of course, what happened was that my oncologist ordered a port, and my medical insurance covered it. I am extremely fortunate that these two factors resulted in my getting a top-of-the-line port. I was amazed at how the port technology had advanced over the years since I first started studying cancer patients. My port was implanted at the top of the right side of my chest, just below my clavicle and just beneath my skin. You could not really see it unless I pulled my arms back a bit, and then the distinct triangle shape appeared. One line from the port fed directly into a large vein directly above my heart. So, when they started my drips, I was looking directly at the fluids entering my body right near my heart.

Throughout my entire treatment experience, I shed a few tears every time they accessed my port. I was so grateful to have the port, which significantly facilitated my treatment experience, but I have a vivid imagination, so every time they set up the lines, drew up blood to make sure that the line was good, and began the process, I thought about what was happening right beneath my skin, right by my heart.

We started the first infusion with some introductions and a review of what the day would likely look like, and I met the infusion team. One principal nurse would be in charge of me, but other nurses on the floor would share tasks as the day proceeded, and at times, more than one nurse would be in room to help verify that each drug was the appropriate drug for me.

The first head of my infusion team was a seemingly incredibly confident, no-nonsense woman, I suspect about fifteen years my junior. She was not so-licitous or chatty, and I recall feeling comforted by her significant display of self-confidence. Given that this time would be the first I was going to offer up my body to the poisons, her demeanor made me feel safe. I believed that if I were to literally fall—which I could not, as I was in a chair—she would be able to catch me.

The process started with the ingestion of two Tylenol and two Benadryl tablets. Next came the monoclonal antibody, rituximab. The nurse had instructed me that I needed to tell them if I felt any reaction to the rituximab as, as noted earlier, it sometimes causes an immune response. The reactions they wanted me to report included fever or chills, skin rash and itching, flushing, nausea, vomiting, headache, tongue or throat swelling, and/or difficulty breathing.

Not surprisingly, I suppose, I drifted off into a restless sleep as the process began due to the combination of not sleeping well the night before because of anxiety and ingesting the two Benadryl tablets. My husband was my support person for the first infusion, and as I wafted for a moment out of this sleep, I mentioned to him that both of my inner ears were very itchy. He asked whether that was something we should report to the nurses. I did not think that it rose to the level of the symptoms I should be reporting, but we decided to tell them anyway. The team immediately sprang into action and halted the infusion. Yes, this symptom was exactly the kind I should report! Since I had already taken the Benadryl, the course of action was to temporarily halt the infusion and then start it back up, but very slowly, to reduce the likelihood of any additional reactions to the monoclonal antibodies. This course of action was successful.

The remaining drugs, except for the Red Devil, were administered via IV bags. The Red Devil was administered by hand by a nurse, still directly into the IV line in my port, but by syringe instead of as an IV drip. This method is called a "push." Given the extreme toxicity of this drug, the nurse administering the push would have to take extra precautions—putting on multiple gowns and gloves—before beginning the procedure. Watching the nurses go through this routine during every outpatient infusion was a harsh reminder that the Red Devil and all the other drugs were not "safe" substances. Every extra glove and gown reminded me that the medical team was trying their best to not come into contact with these fluids.

Confirming Name and Birth Date

As a safety protocol, patients are asked to state their name and birth date before any procedure starts. And I mean *any*—from taking a blood sample, to accessing a port, to administering Tylenol, to changing an IV bag. During a typical infusion appointment, it was not uncommon to be asked to confirm my name and birth date fifteen-plus times over seven hours. Being asked to repeat this information multiple times during one visit could start to get annoying—repeating over and over "Virginia O'Connell, 5/17/64" (I left out the "Adams" for their convenience). While it was a comforting safety measure, it was oddly depersonalizing, as a part of me wanted them to remember who I was! Over time, I offered the information as a learned chant in response to their inquiry, almost transforming it into a sacred plea that the medicine would work. Do you accept this bag of rituximab in an attempt to survive? Virginia O'Connell, 5/17/64, I do.

Limiting Touch

The nursing staff limits their contact with the substances for their own protection, but they also repeatedly disinfect their hands and glove up to protect the cancer patient. As noted before, many chemotherapy drugs leave the patient immunocompromised (see "neutropenia" in the earlier list of side effects). As is the case in many medical settings, contagion control measures are closely followed. As I was sitting there watching them take such care, I appreciated their efforts to not expose me to any infectious substances.

But herein also lay a challenge: I was often scared, especially at the first infusion. Few patients will have experienced any medical procedures quite like what they will experience during their cancer treatments. When I am at my primary care physician's office for bronchitis, I may be anxious, but I am usually not so anxious as to call myself scared. But when you are faced with your possible mortality, and with an understanding that you are going to have to feel much worse before you can feel better, body and psyche want nothing more than to be hugged (direct touch) and comforted. These caretakers are about to drip and push poisons in your body to save your life. As you begin the treatment process, your mind is actively wrestling with this affront to our common concept that medicine makes us feel better. This perception is in part why the staff's display of a combination of competency and kindness is so important. You are unlikely to get to know any individual staff member well since they rotate on and off their work schedules and may or may not overlap with you again. However, if you knew them well enough for them to hug you as you sit there, scared in your chair, then maybe you would also feel more comfortable watching them hook you up to the IV bags. So, in the name of self-protection and contagion control, the smile as they come into the room, the sharing of a joke or anecdote, a really clear explanation of what is happening right now—all of these acts become the needed hugs. When the team successfully establishes that connection, your stress level starts to fall, and you lie back in the infusion chair, ready to begin. It takes an enormous amount of faith to consent, to offer your arm, or your port, up to the needles and tubes and fluids of various colors.

Passing Time and Side Effects

My first infusion took almost seven hours, in part because of the minor allergic reaction I had to rituximab. I was relieved that I did not have any other commitments that day. As noted earlier, over the course of my infusions, I witnessed a number of patients who had to go directly from an infusion to their jobs, and I could not imagine after such a long day how anyone could either physically or mentally do that.

Since we had been warned that the day might be very long, we were encouraged to bring a lunch, snacks, other beverages, and so forth or to plan to buy lunch somewhere in or near the Perelman Center. The infusion center also had a small kitchen stocked with some beverages and snacks. I was so distracted by my anxiety about starting the experience that I did not put much thought into the food we brought that day. We packed a few turkey sandwiches and brought our water bottles.

Once we got home, I wanted to go out for a walk. I had just spent the better part of the past seven hours in an infusion chair, only getting up for short walks to the bathroom and to walk up and down the hallways a bit as the staff changed the different IV bags. I wanted to walk, as I needed to stretch my limbs—I could not remember the last time I had sat for such an extended period of time. While a good portion of my working life is spent sitting at a desk in front of a computer, I have multiple breaks during the day when I move about, especially when I am teaching—lecturing, drawing on the board, interacting with students.

Since I knew that I would very likely start experiencing side effects from treatment, I also wanted to walk before it got harder to walk. I also had a semi-scientific rationale behind wanting to walk: Since I knew that the lymphoma was in my humerus, my pelvic bone, and my femurs, I theorized that walking would help get the drugs deep into my bones. I chuckled to myself as this thought took shape. I recognized that I was actively seeking any way to feel in control of my destiny as the journey began. My husband accompanied me in case I had any reaction to the first treatment.

While it took two weeks to begin losing my hair, I felt other side effects more immediately. The first was extreme fatigue. I suspect that the fatigue was not just from the first infusion but also from the surgery to place my port as well as other pretreatment tests (a cranial MRI, for example). But this fatigue was intense and somewhat indescribable. One of the informational handouts I received from my care team describes this fatigue as "not relieved by rest or sleep," and it was not exaggerating. Once you accept that you will not feel relief from the fatigue, no matter how much you rest or sleep, and once you understand that it is expected and "normal," you adjust to living a life constantly feeling like you need a nap. Nothing helps—not even coffee. I increasingly found myself sitting almost stock-still in my favorite chair in the living room, just sitting, for sometimes up to thirty minutes between such simple activities as putting on a load of laundry or making some lunch. I could not read, could not look at my phone—nothing.

In addition to the fatigue, I also experienced some of the expected gastrointestinal side effects—I certainly experienced nausea. But at this early stage, I was still able to keep my fluids up and enjoyed most meals. Despite the nausea, I did experience a significant, I would even call it extreme, increase in my craving for protein. I even started dreaming about eating protein. Given the (hopefully sizable!) level of cellular destruction from the chemotherapy, the craving seemed scientifically rational. In particular, I craved lox. I did not even need a bagel or cream cheese.

I had hoped that the second infusion would take less time than the first, as they can administer rituximab more quickly once the initial fears of an immune response pass (the allergic reaction is usually limited to the first infusion). But the second outpatient infusion took eight hours due to the sheer number of people being treated that day. A series of minor delays included getting the results from my blood test that morning—which I had to "pass" before infusions could begin—as well as delays getting all my drugs from the pharmacy.

My sister, Mary Kay Adams, was my support person for the second infusion. She is two years older than I and has been my best friend since we shared a bedroom as children. After a career as an actor, she became an ASL (American Sign Language) interpreter. It is amazing how her acting skills inform her signing; she is an incredibly animated and beautiful interpreter. She currently lives in northern New Jersey but did not hesitate for a second in saying that she wanted to come down to be with me.

The bulk of her interpreting work happens at colleges and universities and in medical settings. She has interpreted countless appointments at Memorial Sloan Kettering Cancer Center, the cancer treatment and research institution in the borough of Manhattan in New York City, so she was already extremely familiar with the operation of infusion departments, even though she had never interpreted for someone with primary bone lymphoma. Her familiarity with a typical infusion experience resulted in her coming more prepared for my infusion visit than I could have ever envisaged or accomplished for myself.

She was fully prepared for my drifting off for short naps throughout the day, especially after taking the Benadryl. She arrived with an incredibly varied picnic of different foods. Knowing that at this stage of treatment, some foods might be more tolerated than others, and that the degree of toleration could change daily, she filled her cooler with different proteins, fruits, and snacks. My heart cheered when she showed me two snacks in particular—a cheese Danish from a notable bakery in her area (a favorite of mine since childhood) and the famous "black and white cookie," known to anyone familiar with the New York metropolitan area. Calling the "black and white" a cookie is somewhat misleading, as it more like a flattened vanilla cupcake, half iced with chocolate and half with vanilla frosting or fondant.[37] If you have never tried a black and white, try to find one!

But perhaps the greatest support was my sister's ability to keep my mind and heart engaged. We spent all the time I was not napping talking, reflecting, musing, and laughing, and the hours and the changing IV bags passed quickly. She brought a variety of "white noise" recordings to play while I was napping. She also brought *The Questions Book: 300 Questions to Get People Talking*, by Joe Nyquist, to help us when I might feel a bit overwhelmed by what was happening or when I felt particularly horrible—dealing with extreme nausea, for example.[38] The book is marketed as a way to spark conversations and potentially change outlooks. The questions can be intriguing or silly. My sister would sense my anxiety and suddenly tell me to pick a number between 1 and 300. She would then look up that question, and we would take turns answering. Here are a few examples:

> #17: You're on a road trip and the only place to get anything for lunch is a gas station. What do you buy?

#55: Where are you looking forward to going to visit someday?

#213: What little thing makes you way more happy than it should?

It was comforting to not think about the danger I was in and to think about what I would get to eat from a gas station. It was nice to think optimistically about where I still would like to visit. And it was also nice to think about the little things that still were bringing me joy, such as my vegetable garden growing, my flowering perennials setting some buds, and the nuthatches and chickadees visiting my birdfeeders.

After the second outpatient infusion, my fatigue increased significantly. I was grateful that having my two dogs at home provided not only company and comfort but also motivation to walk every day because the temptation to sit still could become overwhelming. I often did feel better after one of our walks, even though there were times when I would have to sit on a neighbor's front stoop for a few minutes before I could continue. At this stage, despite the fatigue and gastrointestinal discomforts, I still generally felt okay, even though I also felt what I can only describe as a bit beaten up.

Adjusting to Physical Changes

As noted in the previous chapter, I started to lose my hair exactly two weeks after my first infusion. It took a few more weeks to lose all the hair on my head except for a few diffuse strands that refused to give up their hold throughout the entire treatment process. A few weeks later, I also lost essentially all my eyelashes, eyebrows, leg and arm hair, and pubic hair. In anticipation of the loss, my oncologist wrote a prescription for a wig during my first consultation, which I never filled. I think that my fatigue was so extreme so quickly, I could not muster the energy needed to explore this option. I also started my treatment in June, so the summer heat made me less eager to think about donning wigs.

I had heard from some previous cancer patients that to make the inevitable hair loss less traumatic, they shaved their heads before they even began treatment, exerting some control over the process. I will control the timing of the loss, not you, chemotherapy! I was not ready to do the complete shave—as noted, I had not really focused on the reality that I would lose my hair—so I took a middle stance and asked my eldest to give me a short bob. They came over in the afternoon, and we went out to the backyard with some hair scissors and a comb. I wanted to get the cut done outside to make the cleanup as easy as possible. We left my hair in the garden for the birds and squirrels to use for their nests. I was not sure whether any animals would use the hair, but the idea that the cut was not just a loss brought me comfort.

For most of my childhood and adulthood, I have had long hair. As a very young child, my sister and I had "pixie" cuts (very short hair), a popular children's hairstyle in the 1950s and 1960s. While it was easy to care for, I was teased for years about my kindergarten class picture since I ended up looking like an actual pixie (in a green dress with orange flowers, an oversize orange bow, and a broad white collar—classic!). I asked my mother shortly after we got my kindergarten picture if I could possibly grow my hair out, promising to keep it clean and brushed. My request was timely, as the 1970s fashion brought back the popularity of long hairstyles.[1]

While the bob was my compromise, it was also part of what sociologists would call my anticipatory socialization into the cancer patient role.[2] While pursuing my diagnosis, I had seen many cancer patients in the waiting rooms where I was tested, scanned, prodded, and poked. I also knew the typical cancer patient's appearance from my own research and personal experiences with family members: a bald head, an exhausted guise, perhaps a head scarf or hat to provide some coverage. I was starting to physically achieve the "look" and understand more completely my impending deep dive into the sick role. The testing process itself consumed hours of my time—at times a full workday. I started practicing the cancer patient role—filling out forms, following instructions, answering numerous questions, waiting patiently, lying very still in the machines, offering my arm up for another blood sample, interacting with a variety of medical professionals and support staff.

But all this knowledge and anticipation, and my attempt to make the transition gradual, did little to actually ease the distress of my first physical transformation. Shortly after getting the bob, I was struck by my reflection in the storefront windows of my town center, which I first saw out of the corner of my eye as I was out walking my dogs. The person reflected in the glass looked like a stranger. I did not recognize myself without my long hair twisted up on my head. And this question was not about whether I looked "good" or "attractive" with the new short hair; it was fundamentally about whether I looked like *me*. And I became acutely aware that I would soon look even less like me.

Anticipatory Socialization, Resocialization, and Social Interactionism

In Robert K. Merton's work on anticipatory socialization and Erving Goffman's analysis of total institutions, the authors provide frameworks for understanding adult socialization throughout the course of our lifetimes.[2,3] Anticipatory socialization provides us with opportunities to "practice" new roles and the associated appropriate attitudes and behaviors. The new attitudes and behaviors we need to adopt require varying degrees of transformation, from the minor to the major, depending on the demands of the new role. Let us think of a first-time parent. Throughout the pregnancy, the expectant individual and, if applicable, their partner are told by friends and family members that their lives will never be the same once their baby is born since seasoned parents recognize how many aspects of their childless lives changed once they were parents. And the expectation is that you will change your behavior: You will not go out to the movies on a whim, you will eat more balanced meals, you will keep to a more regular schedule. The expectant parent can practice being a new parent in a variety of ways: They can spend time with other people's babies, perhaps babysitting, and they can prepare for their expected role and new demands by setting up a nursery. And each item they purchase signals the particular new demands associated with the care of a newborn—feeding, bathing, stimulating, protecting, and soothing.

Or think of the recent high school graduate heading off to college. Many college students find navigating a sudden increase in "free time" to be a significant challenge, sometimes more so than managing the actual college coursework.[4] Hopefully, college preparation classes have prepared them for greater academic demands, but many students' lives outside school prior to college were scheduled by parents and/or guardians and filled with activities. Trying to create and manage a new schedule on their own leaves many first-year students feeling uncomfortable in their new social role. Greater comfort can be achieved if the student has pre-socialization experiences prior to college where they can practice independent time management, such as sleepaway camps, travel opportunities, and work experiences that require some self-direction.

The greater the distance between the current and the new social role, the greater the discomfort, and the more complex the process of resocialization. In Merton's and Goffman's analyses of military recruits, we see the ways resocialization turns civilians into soldiers. Part of the boot-camp experience involves stripping away all outward signs of your individuality. I cut your hair or narrowly define how you can wear it so that everyone's hair looks similar. I take away your personal clothing and give you common uniforms. You were an individual, but now you are first and foremost a member of a team. You must learn to follow orders without question. I tell you when to wake up and when to go to sleep. I tell you when you can eat. I must take away all the old familiar behaviors and establish new ones to transform you into a soldier.

The role of soldier is demanding, and therefore the transformation process is notoriously extreme and challenging.[5]

People entering prisons undergo similar stripping rituals. You hand over all your personal possessions for inspection. You wear the prison uniform. I tightly control your schedule. I limit the number and kinds of personal items you can possess while incarcerated. I assign you a number in addition to your name.

In both cases, resocialization involves the stripping away of individuality and autonomy. In the case of the soldier, this process is done in the name of preparing recruits for the obligations and functions of the social role. In the case of the prisoner, this stripping functions as punishment.

While these examples of resocialization in total institutions are extreme, we can use these frameworks to examine less extreme examples of resocialization in other social institutions. Becoming a patient in a healthcare setting, especially as an inpatient, also involves stripping rituals. One of the first is removing your clothing and putting on the infamous hospital gown. The primary argument for making patients put on the gown is principally functional: The gown provides the best, most complete access for the physician to the patient's body, free from zippers, tight sleeves, buttons, and so forth. Once the patient is stripped down, a physician can easily and quickly access any part of their body without delays caused by clothing adjustment or removal, and in a healthcare environment where patients are backing up in the waiting room, efficiency is highly prized.

But as sociologists argue, a behavior that might be functional for one person may be dysfunctional for another. The hospital gown leaves patients accessible but also feeling exposed and vulnerable.[6] Even though these gowns are supposedly designed as a one-size-fits-all garment, I, for one, have never had one that I believed fit well at any time in my adult life. During an interaction, the fully clothed doctor wears a white coat that signals authority and prestige, while the half-naked patient desperately tries to make sure that "private parts" are not accidently exposed as the gown slips or opens.

Making the patient strip also removes an important communication device. In his work *The Presentation of Self in Everyday Life*, Goffman examines social interactions between individuals in society by using the imagery of the theater as his framework.[7] Goffman makes an argument similar to Shakespeare's—"All the world's a stage, / And all the men and women merely players."[8] Our clothing functions as our costumes in this elaborate play we call our lives. Our clothing choices are important public ways we present ourselves, communicating significant details about our place in society—our gender identity, our ethnicity, our community, our likes and dislikes, our socioeconomic status, and even our values. In the act of asking us to take off all these signals, like the soldier in training and the incarcerated individual, the doctor standardizes our institutional uniform, stripping away signals that might convey important information in addition to representing core aspects of our self-identities.

George Herbert Mead's concept of social interactionism and Charles Horton Cooley's concept of the looking-glass self provide additional interesting frameworks for thinking about the impact of this stripping ritual on doctor-patient interactions.[9,10] Mead argues that we use symbols and language to create meanings in our interactions with others and that we reflect on how we are perceived by others, potentially altering or modifying our symbols and language if we do not experience a desired response. Mead argues that certain social and power structures can limit and impair an individual's experience when they are denied the ability to characterize themselves.[11] This disempowerment of individual autonomy and expression is the goal when we strip the military recruit and the prisoner of their personal clothing. But is this experience what we want for the patient? Given that the sick patient is already challenged by their illness, what additional experiential burdens result from taking away personal clothing, a mode of expression and communication?

Cooley's looking-glass analysis describes the process by which we form our self-opinions based on our interactions with others. Leigh S. Shaffer summarizes Cooley's argument by defining three key steps:

1. We imagine how we must appear to others in a social situation.
2. We imagine and react to what we feel their judgment of that appearance must be.
3. We develop our sense of self and respond through these perceived judgments of others.[12]

The stripped cancer patient, whose appearance has been standardized, struggles to assess how the medical staff is reacting to their physical appearance, which, once treatment is underway, is often quickly significantly compromised by the side effects of said treatment. Stripped down to a gown, the patient strains to maintain their individual identity, their connection to the social world. As discussed in Chapter 2, the cancer patient often tries to read their physicians' responses and demeanor for any information related to their prognosis. And the patient ponders, "Does my doctor seem pleased or concerned by my appearance? Are they treating me like a potential survivor?"

And it is not only the responses of their physicians; cancer patients spend a great deal of energy trying to read their technicians' responses to their X-rays, scans, reports, and so forth. The technicians performing the various tests have some of the best "poker faces" I have ever seen. They rarely share any of their insights, even though you know that they have insights. They have just performed an ultrasound on your thyroid, your breast, your heart, and they must have a sense from their accumulated experience about whether everything generally looks okay or not. But the final authoritative reading will be made by the radiologist, so they do not say. Conversations with technicians are often stilted and stunted—purposefully terse to protect against an inappropriate release of information. Although this limitation is meant to protect the technician and the patient, it results in unnatural and uncomfortable exchanges.

The cancer patient, therefore, experiences a significant variation of normal social interactions when interacting with medical personnel. My normal communication behaviors do not work. My physicians and other technicians will rely more on reading my blood work and my scans to assess how I am doing than on interacting with me in real time. My "presence" in these social interactions involves not just my physical presence but a separate scientific analysis of my physical components—blood work and scans—that I may or may not understand. I cannot read their reactions to me in real time, especially if we are waiting for test results. If you have ever looked at yourself in a cloudy mirror (for example, an antique mirror), you can appreciate the resulting uneasiness. I cannot clearly decipher how I appear, and I know that others are deliberately trying to avoid reacting to my appearance (since it is by definition incomplete). Therefore, I have an incomplete sense of self and cannot respond. The persistence of the cloudiness leaves the cancer patient feeling unmoored. At times, you are left feeling more uncertain, more "unseen," after a medical appointment than you did before you saw your medical team.

Maintaining a Role for Personal Clothing

During inpatient and outpatient chemotherapy sessions, patients could wear their own clothing as long as it did not impede medical procedures. The staff recommended super comfortable clothing, such as lounge pants and loose tops and T-shirts. My only constraint for my inpatient stays was to make sure that whatever top I was wearing would not interfere with access to my port (on the top right side of my chest) and the lines that would be connected. Before certain tests, such as PET and CT scans, MRIs, and X-rays, there were often additional considerations, such as avoiding clothing with metal components, such as hooks (bras!), zippers, snaps, and so forth. I was also instructed to remove all jewelry, which I was actually unable to do since I could not remove my nose piercing without a special tool (luckily, this inability proved to be a problem only once). I had not focused on the avoidance of metal before my first scans, so I had to change into the dreaded gown. Once I put together an acceptable outfit for these tests, I wore that outfit every time. Since it was unlikely the same technicians would administer a test more than once, I did not worry that I would be judged for repeatedly wearing the same black harem pants with the elephant print.

Based on the preceding analyses and on the work of other researchers, we should consider the benefits of allowing patients to wear personal clothing whenever possible.[13,14] During the doctor-patient interaction, the patient might find significant comfort in being able to silently communicate the messages relayed by their clothing choices. The choices could help physicians understand patients' illness narratives, providing information that could enhance communication, facilitate the process of informed consent, and even help them understand patients' decisions, strengths, and/or limitations. Acknowledgment of a patient's Phillies T-shirt, college or university hoodie, or lounge pants adorned with sketches of dogs provides an opening for the patient to share information about their passions and perspectives. For example, I am not just another cancer patient you are seeing today—I'm a person who loves dogs. When you want information about my level of fatigue, you can ask me about how often I am getting my dogs out for a walk. I can provide objective, concrete information about how I am affected by the treatments that is more meaningful than marking my level of fatigue on a scale from "a little" to "a lot." Personal narratives can also help the physician more fully understand the patient's quality of life.

For one of my outpatient chemotherapy sessions, I purposefully wore my Rose Tree Women's Soccer hoodie, even though I knew that I would be spending the day sitting in an infusion chair and not running around a soccer field. Wearing this shirt helped lighten the weight of the sick role I would be occupying all day. My shirt announced to everyone at the Abramson Cancer Center that I was more than a cancer patient—I was also a middle-age-plus athlete who hoped to play soccer again! By wearing this shirt, I attempted to communicate a role I held other than patient—to communicate strength and hope for the restoration of functioning.

Forced Resocialization from Treatment Effects

While some socialization into the sick role results from behavioral and "uniform" changes enforced by the medical institution, a significant resocialization for cancer patients results from the physical side effects of treatment. As I have shared earlier, cutting my hair short had an immediate significant impact on my self-perception, so it will not be surprising to hear that the loss of the vast majority of my hair had an even greater impact. But some of the changes are deeper than those that just appear on the surface. Your relationship with your entire body can change and morph in unexpected ways. Together, they make it hard for the cancer patient to recognize themselves, using any of their senses.

Hair

My hair started falling out on the evening of July 4, the day before I was scheduled to go to the hospital for my first inpatient infusion. I noticed a sudden but unmistakable change right after I got out of the shower: As I ran my fingers through my hair, I came away with twenty to thirty hairs trapped between my digits. While some cancer patients lose their hair in clumps, mine started and continued as a steady stream of shedding. I started to cry as I looked at my hands. My son was home visiting from Boston, and he came into my bedroom and just held me. Knowing that it would happen and cutting my hair much shorter still did not prepare me for this moment. But then I realized that this change meant that my chemotherapy cocktail was having an effect, and perhaps this loss was a positive sign.

Since I was having trouble facing the loss of my hair, I really had done nothing to prepare myself. Luckily for me, one of my best friends, who is a terrifically talented knitter, began knitting a slouchy beanie for me as soon as she heard about my diagnosis. Fortuitously, she finished the hat on the evening of the Fourth, so I knew that I would be able to bring it with me to the hospital for that first inpatient chemotherapy session. My scalp felt tender, and the incredibly soft steel-blue beanie she knitted provided protection and comfort. I felt bad for the environmental service personnel during that first inpatient stay, and I continued to steadily lose my hair once it began. Every time they came into my room, they were sweeping up strands of my hair. I apologized that I had not anticipated that this loss would happen, and they all told me that they did not mind one bit. I wanted to hug them for their kindness.

Despite being gifted this lovely hat, as my family knows, I do not like hats—basically, I never have (except for the fedora I wore in my early twenties as a fashion statement). I suspect that this dislike is because as a child, I was often sick and forced to wear hats since the theory at that time was that having a "cold head" could get you sick. My dislike of hats, therefore, links back to my dislike of the sick role I often occupied throughout my childhood. Since I have worn my hair long for my entire adulthood, I have never needed hats to keep my head warm. I would twist my hair up, clip it at the top of my head, and be ready to go—warm or cold weather. But once I lost the majority of my hair, I needed some protection for my newly naked scalp to regulate my temperature and to protect my head from sun exposure (R-CHOP therapy renders patients' skin photosensitive—more likely to sunburn). Over the course of my treatment, I primarily relied on three hats—my blue knitted slouchy beanie, a sky-blue baseball cap, and a very wide-brimmed white sun hat with a neck flap that I wore for long walks with my dogs on very sunny days. The wide brim and neck flap of the sun hat protected me from burns on my face and neck, but whenever I wore it, I always felt as though I looked like a beekeeper about to embark on a safari. I laughed every time I put it on and caught my reflection in a window or door.

A few weeks after that July 4, I lost almost all the hair on my head. I say "almost" because throughout the months of treatment, a fairly evenly dispersed light fuzz covered my entire scalp. When the wind blew over my bare head, it tickled, which was an oddly pleasant sensation, even while it reminded me that I had lost my hair. I often wondered what it was about these particular hair follicles that made them immune to the chemotherapy drugs.

As noted earlier, it was not just the hair on the top of my head that I lost: I also lost the vast majority of my eyebrows, eyelashes, leg and arm hair, and pubic hair. The most annoying side effect from losing my eyelashes was that my eyes hurt all the time. They constantly felt dry, and they often watered, which caused my eyeglasses to fog up. My treatment team suggested that I use cold compresses, cold eye masks, and occasionally some soothing eye drops, but the discomfort often interfered with my desire to read or work on the computer.

Any positives to my hair loss? If a single silver lining to hair loss existed during treatment, it was that I sprouted no chin hairs! Since my mid-thirties, I have groomed the sporadic thicker chin hairs that emerged as my body began producing less estrogen. By the time I was diagnosed, plucking a few stray hairs had become part of my daily grooming routine. The chin hairs never bothered me, but they were clearly affected by the chemotherapy drugs. This overall hair loss reduced the time and attention I had to spend on grooming!

Smell and Scent

My sense of smell and my experience of my own body odor were significantly affected by the chemotherapy. This impact, therefore, also affected my sense of taste. This effect is not surprising since a fraction of the receptor cells in our noses and taste buds comprise quickly renewable cells, and since many chemotherapy drugs target quickly dividing cells, some patients will lose a portion of their smell receptors and taste buds during treatment.[15,16]

I have always been very sensitive to odors, reporting a greater and deeper appreciation of or reaction to smells than did other people around me. This sensitivity has always enriched my enjoyment of the natural world and has served me well in my enjoyment of cooking. For example, when teaching my children to cook, I often told them to rely on the smell of certain dishes to help decide whether they were seasoned correctly or ready. So, chemotherapy's impact on my sense of smell, while not dire, was very personally disconcerting. While I was walking my dogs during those months of treatment, the summer grass, Crum Creek, and the flowering plants smelled less enchanting, less alive. While I still enjoyed cooking, I had to avoid certain foods that suddenly did not smell familiar or appetizing.

This experience also underscored for me the degree to which until my diagnosis, I had tracked my own well-being based on my odor. The fact that I no longer fully recognized my own "smell" was disorienting and, in short, unpleasant. I did not smell like myself—another way in which this experience diminished my sense of self. I not only visually was a stranger but also smelled like a stranger. As reported by other cancer patients (extensively on blogs and social media sites), my personal scent was infiltrated by underlying tones of sharp chemicals.[17] This change is not unexpected since the body will expel the chemotherapy drug waste through a variety of means—urine, stool, tears, and sweat.[18] This smell was not the sharp chemical smell associated with detergents and cleaning products but more akin to the chemical odor you experience when working in or walking through science labs (think back to any "chem lab" experience you had in school).

I also experienced one significant change in the way that I expelled sweat: In addition to all the normal spots, I started sweating from my cheeks. Before treatment, when sweating cranially, like most people I know, I would sweat from my brow/hairline, the top of my lip, and my neck, but once I started chemotherapy, I began sweating from my cheeks. It was an extremely odd sensation that became a permanent change. Apparently, this change can result from stress or anxiety. This particular odd change has not been linked to R-CHOP therapy.

If you consume any advertising in the United States, you learn fairly quickly about Americans' obsession with controlling perspiration and odors—body and household. Americans shower more than many Europeans do, but not as much as our Mexican neighbors.[19] We are encouraged—to the detriment of the health of our own skin—to shower daily, to use strong antiperspirants and deodorants, to use fragrance-enhanced soaps, laundry detergents, cleaning products, and air fresheners. We so frequently strip away our natural oils, we are forced to use moisturizing creams, with about 69% of the U.S. population using supplemental creams and lotions.[20] The clean-smelling body (free from any offending suggestion of sweat) and the clean-smelling home are normative idealized states. Fresh breath is also highly valued. Studies estimate that 95%–98% of Americans brush their teeth at least once per day, 93% of adults wear deodorant when seeing other people, and about 85% shower every day.[21] Consequently, emitting the scent of a high-school or college chemistry lab does not fall within the norms of acceptable smells.

Americans started using deodorants around 1888 and using a combination of deodorants and antiperspirants in the early 1900s, but an aggressive marketing campaign against sweat and body odor began between 1912 and 1919. In its early use to block perspiration, aluminum chloride had to be suspended in acidic base compounds and, therefore, could cause skin irritation in the armpits and stain clothing. To overcome people's intolerance of these undesirable side effects, advertisements launched linking female sweat to a woman's inability to attract and keep a man. In the early 1900s, sweating was still considered a display of masculinity and, therefore, not a problem for men. But when the early makers of deodorants and antiperspirants realized that by not also marketing to men, they were missing half of their potential customer base, sweating and the smell of sweat for men were also identified as problems to be controlled, especially for the professional man in an office.[22] What had been normative and in fashion became unacceptable and unfashionable.

Our tolerance for and acceptance of certain smells depend on the context.[23] Humans tend to pay little attention to the smells common in their normal environments, but our senses are heightened by new and changing smells. The city dweller visiting the countryside is likely to be far more sensitive to the smell of farm animals than is the farm worker, and the farm worker is likely to be far more sensitive to the smells of vehicular exhaust when visiting the city than is their city friend. Very few smells are inherently unpleasant for humans, although one such odor is ammonia, which, as is theorized, helps us avoid its toxic impacts.[24]

The smells of our social worlds, therefore, are socially constructed—dependent on cultural norms, historical contexts, and market forces defining fads and fashion (florals might be the current preference, but next season, perhaps it will be citrus). The standards, however, do form an experiential basis on how we present ourselves in our world and how we interact with others in that world. Evidence suggests that even when our natural smells are masked by deodorants and soaps, we are able to unconsciously assess other people's emotional states based on their smells.[25] Chemotherapy disrupts patients' olfactory experience of their world. They lose important ways to assess their own well-being, to present themselves appropriately to others through their scent, and to effectively assess the scents of others around them. Collectively, these losses contribute to their overall sense of discomfort and unease.

Taste

As previously noted, chemotherapy also affects the cells that compose our taste buds. But beyond the direct impact on my taste buds, the impact on my nasal receptor cells alone would have diminished my sense of taste. Most of us can recall a time when a head cold made our food taste bland. While the taste buds decipher whether the food we are eating is sweet, sour, salty, bitter, or savory, our sense of smell is what allows us to decipher the difference between a raspberry and a strawberry.[26]

In addition to my metallic body odor, after starting chemotherapy, I experienced a constant metallic aftertaste. This terrible aftertaste was always worst when I was taking prednisone. This sensation significantly interfered with my enjoyment of many foods and beverages. I will highlight two of the most disappointing impacts:

- **Coffee:** My beloved coffee. I could not sense the depth of flavor—all coffee tasted rather flat and uninteresting. I really missed enjoying a good cup of coffee. But, as noted earlier, even a good cup of coffee could not touch my incredibly deep fatigue.
- **Sweets:** I would not describe myself as someone with a sweet tooth, but before treatment, I generally enjoyed sweets. During treatment, I basically lost my enjoyment of sweet items. If I had something sweet—a piece of candy, a pastry, a slice of pie—I only ever wanted a few bites. Any more, and the sensation of the sweet food in my mouth became unpalatable. It is challenging to describe. I could still taste "sweet," but it became unwanted.

While coffee and sweets became unpleasant, other tastes became more pleasant, with some becoming nothing short of cravings. The most extreme craving was for protein, so much so that I often dreamed of eating protein. I suspect that this desire was a direct response to the extent of cellular death—my body was craving protein to repair the damage to my body. On more than one occasion, I sat down and consumed 8 ounces of lox at a single sitting. I often ate it plain or with a little cream cheese—no bagel, crackers, or toast. I also more than once ate a small jar of herring with sour cream. Other favorite protein sources included turkey kielbasa and sliced deli turkey breast, again, eaten without any accompanying carbohydrates.

My drink of choice was consistently unsweetened iced tea with a splash of lemonade. The one sweet drink that I often inexplicably craved was mango juice. Mangos are one of my favorite fruits, but I'm not sure why mango juice suddenly became the desired form.

The last two food highlights are cucumbers with sour cream and vinegar-based items. I could eat cucumbers and sour cream no matter how nauseated I felt. I also consistently enjoyed pickles, olives, vinegar-based salad dressings, and pickled ginger.

While I was lucky to find foods that I consistently enjoyed, it would be negligent for me to gloss over the degree of loss that changing tastes and tolerances can have on patients. Our food preferences reflect far more than our nutritional needs; the foods we prepare and enjoy are, like our clothing choices, reflections of our traditions, social experiences, communities, cultural histories. My references to lox, herring, and kielbasa reflect the Jewish and Polish influences on my family's food choices. In American society, we use the term *comfort foods* to define foods that we consume to manipulate our emotional states or feelings.[27] We recognize the ritualistic significance of certain foods, from birthday cakes to a traditional Thanksgiving turkey. We cherish and celebrate occasions to share meals with our loved ones and friends. A common act of caring is to make a meal for someone.

All these meaningful acts of consuming food can be interrupted by cancer treatments. Formerly reliable comfort foods might become unpalatable or unmanageable.[28] Due to a combination of being immunocompromised and constantly nauseated, the patient may be unable to participate in holiday meals. They are impaired from fully participating in normal social interactions, even when they are between treatments. And the act of caring that family and friends might offer—bringing over a meal—may not provide the desired comfort and support. A friend of mine with ovarian cancer recalled the numerous meals made by neighbors during her treatment that her husband ate alone, as she could not tolerate many of the meals since her nausea was so persistent. She felt awkward about not being able to enjoy these gifts of friendship. After learning about my diagnosis, another friend who was ten years past her experience with breast cancer gifted me a variety of lovely teas, saying that she was pretty confident that I would at least be able to tolerate tea throughout my treatment, and she was right—I drank pots of those teas.

Skin and Nails

For a good portion of my life, I have had keratosis pilaris, primarily on my upper arms and calves. "Keratosis pilaris is a common, harmless skin condition that causes dry, rough patches and tiny bumps, usually on the upper arms, thighs, cheeks or buttocks. . . . Keratosis pilaris results from the buildup of keratin—a hard protein that protects skin from harmful substances and infection. The keratin forms a scaly plug that blocks the opening of the hair follicle. Usually many plugs form, causing patches of rough, bumpy skin."[29] This skin variant is normal. The condition affects 50%–80% of adolescents and about 40% of adults.[30] The condition first appeared when I was a child. It is sometimes colloquially referred to as "chicken skin" since the skin bears some resemblance to the plucked skin of the chicken you purchase at the grocery store.[31] I was sometimes teased for my bumpy skin as a child. The condition magically disappeared as I entered adolescence—a more sensitive time for being the target of body-teasing—but returned after the birth of my first child, when I was twenty-eight. Knowing that it was a normal variant, I have never been concerned about treating it. It causes me no discomfort. There are no fully effective treatments. The patches tend to appear bumpier when the skin is dry, so people who want to diminish the bumpy appearance will use lotions or, sometimes, chemical peels. It often becomes less noticeable during hotter, more humid times of the year, and some sun exposure makes the skin look smoother. But the only possible treatment suggested by my dermatologist was using whatever skin lotion I liked best, as he was not supportive of harsher chemical treatments, such as peels or lotions containing salicylic acid.

But there was one problem with this advice: I really, really, *really* do not like the feeling of lotions and creams on my skin. I never have. This dislike has been a problem since my skin gets terribly dry during the winter. My hands get so dry that they will frequently crack and bleed, and yet I still find it hard to use even the most gentle, least greasy skin creams. I have tried every cream out there, and I've tried applying the cream at night, hoping that I would tolerate the feeling better while asleep, but alas, this trick never worked. The result? I have rarely tried any serious intervention to make my patches of keratosis pilaris look less bumpy.

Remarkably, one of the side effects of the chemotherapy was that my keratosis pilaris disappeared. Based on the conversations I had with my medical team and my dermatologist, this change was likely due to the chemotherapy I received as an inpatient, methotrexate, since low doses of the drug (unlike the high doses I received) are used to treat some dermatological conditions, including psoriasis. I noticed that the patches disappeared a few weeks into treatment. I searched online to see whether other cancer patients had noticed this side effect, and sure enough, I was not the first person to experience it. Clearly, infusing your body with very high doses of a toxic chemical that can do significant damage to your kidneys and liver in the name of smoother skin is not a trade-off anyone should be willing to make. But for the first time since my late twenties, my skin was very smooth without the use of creams and lotions. (Spoiler: The keratosis pilaris returned a few months after I had completed chemotherapy.)

Though the keratosis pilaris disappeared, my dry skin did not. Since chemotherapy often leaves you immunocompromised, cancer patients are encouraged to practice very frequent handwashing and bathing routines to avoid getting sick during treatment. As a result, during my summer of treatment, my skin was even drier than it typically is. The chemotherapy also sometimes produced blisters on my hands. My eldest did suggest an ointment that I could tolerate during therapy that worked well and is fragrance-free—Aquaphor. I still used it sparingly when needed, but I was glad to find something I could tolerate.

A number of my friends who had undergone chemotherapy had warned me that treatment would affect my fingernails, rendering them dry and brittle. Similar to my lack of concern about my bumpy skin, I have never paid much attention to my nails. I can count the number of manicures I have gotten over the course of my lifetime. My nails have always grown well—fast, strong, white tips—but given the amount of time I spend gardening and cooking, and the resulting amount of handwashing I do when engaged in these activities, spending time and money on my nails did not make sense. I shape my nails as they get long, but I never fret when they break. Remarkably, my nails never seemed affected by chemotherapy. They continued to grow and remained strong and white. I would sometimes just marvel at their resilience. I have no idea why they were never affected.

Loss of Self

Collectively, these changes significantly recast the individual into a new social role—that of the cancer patient. Resocialization occurs as a result of adapting to the institutional demands of the patient role, but some resocialization is also the direct result of the treatments. Depending on the degree of impact on the patient's body, changes in appearance as well as on smell and taste can leave the patient unrecognizable to themselves. The image in the mirror is a stranger. I may be unable to present myself in my familiar ways to the world, as my hair may be gone, my clothes restricted, my skin and nails changed. And the way I sense my world is also radically diminished and altered. I emit an odd chemical smell, and the world itself smells unfamiliar and bland. The loss of so many familiar ways of presenting to and consuming the world is destabilizing when the individual is already facing a potentially lethal illness. Kathy Charmaz describes this situation as the "loss of self" for patients who are not just experiencing the deleterious effects of treatment but seeing their self-images crumble.[32] Recognition of the patient's illness narrative is incomplete without the recognition of this impact. Patients begin treatment with the hope that all of these losses are temporary: The hair will return, the sense of smell will stabilize, the metallic aftertaste will pass. The costs, though intense, will be worth the benefit—getting into remission. They hold on to this hope while they also recognize that they are unlikely to ever be quite the same. The journey is likely to be long and brutal, and some of the losses will probably be permanent.

Role Strain and Fatigue
with a Capital "F"

As the newly diagnosed cancer patient adopts the sick role, they might be released from some of the obligations of their normal social roles, such as employee or parent, but rarely does the individual relinquish all their social roles during treatment. The demands of cancer treatment regimens vary considerably. The National Cancer Institute lists ten common forms of treatment: biomarker testing, chemotherapy, hormone therapy, hyperthermia, immunotherapy, photodynamic therapy, radiation therapy, stem cell transplant, surgery, and targeted therapy.[1] These therapies are used in various combinations to treat forty common cancer sites.[2] And the available arsenal of drugs includes more than six hundred individual medications, chemotherapy and/or immunotherapy cocktails, and vaccines to manage side effects.[3] Treatment regimens generally last for three to six months for chemotherapy, while other treatment regimens and combined regimens can last for a year or more.[4] Patients with advanced forms of lung cancer, colorectal cancer, ovarian cancer, and some types of lymphoma are increasingly being treated with maintenance therapies after their initial treatment regimens to help keep the cancer from recurring or to stop the progression and spread of any remaining cancer. Maintenance therapies can include a combination of drugs or hormones, immunotherapy, or targeted therapy and may be taken for years after the initial treatment.[5]

Patients receiving chemotherapy typically have breaks of two to six weeks between infusions to allow the body to recover from each treatment—blood counts, for example, need to rebound before the next dose is given.

While cancer treatments might consume substantial amounts of time over the course of weeks, months, and even years, unlike institutionalized populations, cancer patients regularly move in and out of medical institutions between treatments. While the sick role might come to dominate their identity, especially in light of the physical changes caused by treatment, they might be unwilling and/or unable to relinquish their other social roles. For example, as noted in Chapter 2, the financial burden of treatment might force the individual to continue working, even if the patient finds this burden to be excruciating. Maintaining other social roles while also managing the extreme demands of the sick role will likely lead to role strain and role conflict, and these conflicts are exasperated by treatment fatigue.

Role Strain and Role Conflict

Sociologists use the term *role strain* to describe situations when people find it hard to fulfill the responsibilities associated with their roles in society.[6] The strain may result from wider institutional demands (such as a newly expanded list of role obligations) or from an individual's own temporary limitations (such as an acute illness) that render them incapable of fulfilling the role to their normative level. The term *role conflict* refers to conflicting demands between different roles.[7] Many of us experienced role strain as a result of the COVID-19 pandemic. Roles that might have already been demanding became so much more demanding due to pandemic restrictions and accommodations. Teachers and instructors had to quickly learn new methods of teaching online, straining their already demanding social roles. Students had to adjust to learning through a computer screen. Working parents with school-aged children experienced role strain and role conflict, as they had to continue fulfilling their employment demands while also providing supervision of their now homebound children. They also experienced role conflict, as their parenting roles conflicted with their expanding "teacher" roles during the average school day. While pre-pandemic, parents might have filled some "teaching" roles, such as seeing that homework got completed, they now spent more time and energy on ensuring that their children were engaged in online learning. As a parent, an individual might want to comfort their pandemic-stressed child, but simultaneously, as the new school-day supervisor, they might need to enforce online attendance.

The cancer patient experiences role strain and role conflict throughout their treatment. The side effects affect the patient's physical ability to continue to fulfill their normal social roles when they are between treatments, and the accumulated fatigue often increases this strain over time. The sick role conflicts with all the patient's pre-cancer social roles. In addition to the impairment of the individual's physical ability, there are the added demands made by medical institutions to get tested, receive treatments, attend appointments, and so forth. And medical institutions, by the nature of their organizational demands, constrain patients' flexibility, which could potentially lessen some of the strain and conflict. While the "9 to 5, Monday through Friday" working cancer patient might benefit from weekend appointments and treatments, these are often limited in availability. Patients instead need to conform to the institutional scheduling demands of their medical teams.

The cancer patient might also find it difficult to expect or request accommodations for their role conflicts when they are between treatments. This difficulty results from the normative social pressure to present as functional and competent in public and the lack of a sick-role uniform that could signal the need for modifications. For example, the patient may lose their hair, which could signal to others their sick-role status, but still choose for their own comfort and for the comfort of those around them to wear a wig or a scarf to lessen the shock of the physical transformation. One study found that 84% of patients being treated for breast cancer at a medical center chose to wear a wig during treatment.[8] The patient might also find it challenging to describe the fatigue they feel as a side effect of treatment. While I have discussed the positive functions of wearing your own clothing during treatment, the lack of the "patient gown" or other similar uniform may signal that no accommodations are wanted or needed, even when they might be desperately needed.

But maintaining some normative social roles during treatment has its benefits, even if patients struggle with diminished performance and role strain and conflict. As Stephen R. Marks argues, it is too limited to view human activity—that is, fulfilling our roles—as primarily or exclusively draining.[9] Social and physical activity produce and consume energy. Wearing personal clothes, donning wigs and scarves, going off to work, gardening and preparing meals—all can keep the patient who is facing the possibility of their own mortality vitally connected to the world, thereby lifting their mood, energizing their bodies and minds, and providing some solace for their anxiety. Participation in the social world can provide much-needed hope and distraction from the extraordinary demands of treatment.

Flexibility can be the key for minimizing the strain and conflict that the patient might feel. Some days, they might find that they are very functional, while other days, not at all. The solution might be finding the most effective ways to let patients communicate their sometimes-unpredictable levels of functioning and to provide them with sometimes-unpredictable additional support.

Extreme Fatigue

Chemotherapy fatigue is not a well-understood phenomenon, even though about 85%–90% of patients will report experiencing fatigue at some time during their treatment and cite it as one of the most distressing side effects of cancer treatment.[10,11] There are numerous probable causes, but the relative weight of these factors is uncertain:[12]

- Cancer cells releasing proteins that cause fatigue
- Chemotherapy agents destroying fast-growing cells (fatigue can be the response to the body's need to repair the damage)
- Chemotherapy protocols causing anemia, which can cause fatigue
- Chronic pain
- Anxiety, stress, or depression
- Lack of sleep
- Inadequate nutrition, especially from treatment-induced nausea and vomiting
- Lack of or decreased exercise
- Hormonal changes

For those receiving chemotherapy, the body excretes the chemotherapy drugs about forty-eight hours after each infusion, so the fatigue is not from the continued action of the drugs in the body. Certain drugs are more strongly linked to reports of fatigue. Vincristine (derived from the periwinkle plant) was a main culprit of fatigue among the drugs in my cocktail.

I was not fully prepared for the increasing fatigue over the course of my treatment experience. While I certainly experienced fatigue after the first infusions, it became more persistent and extreme with each additional infusion. I had established some post-infusion routines after my first few outpatient and inpatient infusions to deal with what I knew were going to be the immediate impacts of treatment for a couple of days, but about a month and a half into the process, there was no way to predict the days when I could hope to feel okay and have some energy and the days when I could barely get out of a chair. Not having the ability to predict my energy levels was incredibly frustrating, especially since I was trying to maintain some of my social roles between treatments. As I already shared, I did take a leave of absence from my work as a college professor for a semester, but I was still trying to maintain my social roles as partner to my spouse, mother to my adult children, caretaker of my dogs, neighbor, and friend. Some of the daily duties I tried to fulfill when I was home between treatments included shopping and preparing meals, walking the dogs at least two miles a day, running needed errands, taking care of the yard and garden, and performing other household tasks, such as laundry. But as time passed, even taking care of a few of these tasks became increasingly challenging.

I would plan to take my dogs to the John Heinz National Wildlife Refuge at Tinicum[13] for a walk, or putter in the garden, or run a few errands, only to wake up from a full night's sleep and barely have the energy to get up and get dressed. Too many times to count, I opened my eyes in the morning, felt the crushing weight of the fatigue, and just sobbed. I often felt as though I was not really awake, and I was aware that if I closed my eyes, I could fall asleep in a heartbeat. As someone who had never required much sleep and who had always had trouble falling asleep, this feeling was foreign and uncomfortable. The warning against operating "heavy machinery" that I have read on medicine and alcohol labels all my life corporeally now made sense. When I was under the fog of post-infusion fatigue, I would never have gotten behind the wheel of a car. I so wanted to continue to participate in my life, especially in the joyful aspects, such as my walks with my dogs in nature, my garden, cooking for family and friends—laundry, not so much—but I could barely raise my head off the pillow or my bottom off the couch.

And the number of days between treatments when I felt crushed by fatigue grew with each infusion. I could spend a whole day feeling like a cranky child who needed a nap and often took multiple naps. The fatigue also affected my mood, so in addition to crankiness, I felt quite despondent, and my current medical condition, its treatment protocol, and the general state of the world seemed unbearably heavy. When I felt this way, the temptation to just sit and weep was powerful, and sometimes I let myself do just that. A good cry was occasionally incredibly cathartic. Other times, moving was the best remedy, and I could consistently count on one of my pups nudging my hand when they wanted to let me know it was time for a walk. But even when I managed to get out the door, I could not always complete my task. I recall one particular walk where after walking about one mile, I literally had to sit down and ended up sitting on a neighbor's stoop. As I sat there, holding my dogs' leashes, tears started to flow, and I felt embarrassed while simultaneously wishing that someone would come along, scoop me up into their arms, and carry me back home. I rarely carry my cell phone with me when I am out with the dogs, as I treasure this time to disconnect from technology, but as I sat on that stoop, unable to call my husband or a friend, I thought that perhaps I should start carrying my phone with me, at least while I was in treatment.

Being a "Good Patient"

Treatment for the cancer patient often requires periods of extensive interaction with medical professionals. Unlike basic pharmaceutical interventions, where the patient can take pills during prescribed times during the day, alone or perhaps through the periodic injection, getting scans, X-rays, and chemotherapy and/or radiation therapy requires the devotion of extensive time, coordination of schedules with professional and support personnel, and numerous interactions with schedulers, phlebotomists, nursing assistants, nurses, radiology technicians, surgical staff (for original biopsies and the possible implantation and removal of ports), and oncologists. All these encounters are framed by a set of interactional expectations. Failing to fulfill the normative expected script of the interaction can leave the patient and the medical personnel feeling angry, frustrated, uncomfortable, and/or uneasy.

What Makes a "Good Doctor"?

Each professional medical occupational category has some unique set of expected skills and traits, even though they share many traits. Sociologists recognize the work and experience of physicians as having a special set of rights, responsibilities, and features associated with their professional work. One of the core features is the physician's specialized body of knowledge. This body is so vast and specialized that the profession is given autonomy over the training and licensing process, a significant amount of self-regulation, and, subsequently, high status in society.[1] We give physicians access to our bodies that we do not give to others. They can cut into our flesh, prescribe poisons (in well-defined, nonlethal doses), and touch every part of our body, even places typically reserved for touch by our romantic partners. Given the chasm between their specialized knowledge and the typical patient's lay understandings about anatomy and medicine, the physician-patient relationship is based on deep trust. We trust that they have our best interests at heart in this powerful and unique fiduciary role. They deal with people when they are often in particularly vulnerable states because of their illness or injury. And their expert knowledge and high status, coupled with the patient's hopefully temporary incapacitation, casts them into significant positions of power. This power extends beyond the power exercised during a physician-patient interaction to power over the culture and operation of medical institutions.

Given these rights and responsibilities, what qualities do we look for in our doctors? The answer might depend on whether we are asking physicians or asking patients. Based on the selection process for medical school, the profession unmistakably values academic excellence, demonstrated by high undergraduate GPAs, especially in the natural sciences, as well as a demonstrated commitment to the profession through a variety of shadowing and volunteer experiences.[2] The demand for academic excellence reflects the deep and vast body of knowledge that students must master during medical school. High GPAs signal the innate abilities and habits needed for an even-more-demanding curriculum. The demonstration of a deep vocational calling to the profession through certain extracurricular experiences attempts to measure the psychological fitness of the individual to hold immense power over people's bodies and lives. This demonstrated sacrifice signals that this applicant's motivations are genuine and honorable. But meeting these demands is not easy. They require sufficient resources so that students ideally do not have to earn an income during their undergraduate years. College students who must work to earn income by default have less time that they can devote to master the premedical curriculum and to pursue shadowing and volunteer experiences. In 2017, more than 50% of matriculating medical-school students came from families who were at or above 80% of the income bracket in the United States.[3] And since income is correlated with race, these application demands decrease the chance that Black and Hispanic/Latino applicants will successfully apply. For example, in 2019, only 8.4% of medical-school matriculants were Black, even though they represent 13.6% of the general population. Even more striking is that among matriculants, 6.2% were Hispanic/Latino, even though they represent 18.5% of the general population.[4,5]

Physicians might differentially rank the importance of their professional skills depending on their specialty and their stage of career. Early in training, it is not surprising to learn that medical students and residents rank their technical and knowledge-based competence as the most important trait they can demonstrate, since these skills are continuously measured by their instructors.[6] More seasoned primary care physicians might recognize that kindness and empathy are as important as, if not at times more important than, a complete fund of medical knowledge since only by meeting the patient where they are in their illness experience can the physician understand their patient's lived realities—their resources and limitations—and prescribe realistic treatment protocols.[6]

But there are cases when physicians and patients will trade a good bedside manner for an extreme display of competence and confidence by their physician. Surgeons across surgical specialties are notoriously stereotyped as being "arrogant bastards" with terrible or limited displays of kindness and empathy.[7] We can muse over the reasons why it takes a significant amount of arrogance to be a surgeon. The surgeon must be confident enough to cut into human flesh, to literally hold someone else's life in their hands. They must control their own fatigue and maintain functioning at the height of their skill for the entire duration of a surgical procedure.[8] They must make patients trust that they can successfully operate on them, so patients want to see their surgeons display extreme confidence. But the extreme confidence and arrogance displayed by the surgeon would likely not be tolerated if displayed by the pediatrician.

When patients are asked to identify the qualities that make a good physician, they report a combination of clinical competence and good interpersonal communication skills.[9] Given the gulf between lay and medical knowledge, and given that patients are often in very vulnerable states, the quality of the physician's communication skills demonstrates two key pieces of information to the patient: vital clinical competency and genuine care and concern for the patient's illness state, thereby showing the physician's acceptance of fiduciary responsibility. Patients want their doctors to listen to their stories in part because they want to influence the physician's opinion of them and establish a good doctor-patient relationship.[10] And the patient wants to trust their physician.[11]

What Makes a "Good Patient"?

Much of the discussion by the medical profession about what makes a good patient has centered for decades on patients' levels of compliance with pre-scribed treatments—the more compliant, the better the patient—especially since noncompliance significantly lowers the effectiveness of medical inter-ventions.[12] The loss of effectiveness can lead to treatment failures, progression of disease, hospitalizations, and lost productivity. Suboptimal medication ad-herence has been estimated to cost the U.S. healthcare system between $100 billion and $229 billion annually.[13] While strict compliance is by definition hard to measure when patients are often taking their medications and/or fol-lowing other medical instructions outside the watchful eye of a medical in-stitution, some researchers have estimated that poor compliance is expected in 30%–50% of all patients across conditions and severity of disease states.[14]

A good patient is someone who acknowledges their physician's authority and expertise. Compliance with the prescribed treatment is itself an act of acknowledged authority. Compliance also illustrates that the patient is suc-cessfully adopting Talcott Parsons's sick role, which requires that they seek and follow the advice of legitimate medical practitioners.[15] Through a variety of forums, articles, and blogs, physicians share other traits of good patients: They should show interest in their care, have enough knowledge to have some basic understanding about their condition and treatment, be respectful and appreciative, be manageable (that is, not overly demanding), and present med-ical conditions that are challenging and interesting, but not too obscure, self-inflicted, or resulting from social forces outside the control of medical insti-tutions, such as poverty, abuse, and other forms of social violence.[6,16,17,18,19,20]

Bad patients present an opposite composite of traits from the good pa-tient: They are deemed responsible for their ailments, have little knowledge or understanding of their illness, and are generally behaviorally difficult.[17]

Compliance for the cancer patient begins when they show up for their timed and spaced appointments. Since many successful cancer treatments depend on the well-regulated administration of chemotherapy drugs and/or radiation, skipping a treatment appointment can result in failed control of cancer progression, increased morbidity, and even death.

As long as this minimum requirement is met, when a patient is receiving treatment in the outpatient or inpatient unit, compliance is enforced by the treatment team. They directly administer the required dosage of the medica-tions, so patients cannot mess up the process. But cancer patients may or may not follow instructions for prescribed behaviors between treatments, and this area is where they may be noncompliant. Between treatments, patients are instructed to keep well hydrated, avoid getting sick (especially if treatment has rendered the patient immunocompromised), maintain a healthy diet, and stay as active as possible. As the fatigue and nausea from treatment grow, and as financial pressures might require going to work and getting exposed to others who could be sick, cancer patients might find it increasingly hard to be compliant.

What Makes a Good Doctor-Patient Relationship?

A good doctor-patient relationship results when the physician and the patient each successfully adopt the scripts identified earlier. The physician is competent and genuinely caring. The patient is knowledgeable enough, active in their care, appreciative, and compliant. But what factors will facilitate their effective communication and the development of genuine trust, kindness, and empathy?

Émile Durkheim's concept of mechanical solidarity can help us explore this question.[21] Durkheim defines mechanical solidarity as the social connection we feel with others based on similarities. The more overlap in our characteristics, behaviors, and experiences, the more, he argues, we feel connected to others, based on the assumption that these traits and activities also signal that we share common values and beliefs. Sharing a common language, a base vocabulary, and some social experiences, such as general area of residence, arts, and culture, provides the foundation for engendering mechanical solidarity, which facilitates communication and helps establish trust from a sense of familiarity and comfort.

Studies have shown that shared race between physicians and patients facilitates communication and the assessment of connection and empathy and leads to higher patient satisfaction scores.[22] This result comes from not only facilitating communication but also controlling against implicit bias, especially in cases where the physician is White and the patient is non-White. For example, a study at Stanford showed that Black physicians wrote significantly better and more detailed notes on their Black patients than did their White colleagues.[23] But we have already identified barriers in the selection of medical-school matriculants that impede the profession's ability to better diversify its practitioner population, meaning that the profession cannot currently accommodate race matching, nor will it anytime soon. But the importance of improving communication and limiting the dangerous impacts of bias cannot be understated since studies also show that matching physicians and patients by race has a significant impact on decreasing patients' mortality risk.[24]

While matching physicians and patients on demographic characteristics may increase the effectiveness of the doctor-patient encounter, we can also talk more broadly about the benefit of shared cultural capital in privileging some patients over others in their navigation of the illness experience. Pierre Bourdieu defines *cultural capital* as the set of skills, tastes, mannerisms, credentials, clothing, and so forth that one adopts as being part of a particular social class.[25] Patients who have higher levels of education and, subsequently, higher literacy levels have an advantage when it comes to communication and comprehension of their diagnosis and treatment. Therefore, they are better equipped to demonstrate interest in their care. The closer the patient is to their physician's social class, the more adept they are likely to be in confidently communicating with all staff members in a medical institution. They are better able to advocate for themselves and more readily access various support systems/programs. Shared mannerisms, ways of speaking, and dress reflexively increase the bond between the physician and patient.

Factors that increase the effectiveness of communication between physicians and patients also increase our confidence that this relationship is ethical, especially in the context of assessing genuine informed consent and autonomy. As noted earlier, the good patient is a compliant patient, but the word *compliance* carries a negative, passive connotation. More ideal is the patient who can to some degree comprehend their physician's assessment of their condition and treatment plan, who then freely and without duress agrees with this assessment and then actively participates in the treatment protocol. This scenario is less one of strictly complying and more one of sharing and accepting proposed actions.[26] The ability of the patient to actively engage in dialogue with their physician allows the physician to make recommendations based on clinical expertise without unduly influencing the patient's decision and allows the patient to communicate possible hurdles and challenges in adhering to the treatment plan—in essence, an enhanced concept of autonomy.[27]

But while we can enumerate the demographic and cultural capital factors that facilitate communication and reinforce the expression of genuine autonomy, the reality remains that as of 2021, only 14.4% of adults in the United States over the age of twenty-five had completed an advanced degree, such as a master's degree, professional certification, or doctorate, implying that only a small proportion of the total patient base has the educational skills needed to fully experience this enhanced autonomy.[28] Therefore, we might argue that the medical profession and their institutions must continue to identify ways to facilitate and enhance communication and patients' active participation in their encounters in light of the basically insurmountable gulf between physicians' and patients' knowledge bases. When communication breaks down and desired outcomes are not achieved, clinical failures due to noncompliance can be reinterpreted as medical errors.[29]

Punishing the "Bad Patient"

The dueling concepts of "good" and "bad" patients, coupled with the power that medical practitioners hold in medical institutions, suggest that good patients might be "rewarded" and bad patients "punished," despite physicians' ethical obligation to "provide care to all who need it. . . . It is illegal for a physician to refuse services based on race, ethnicity, gender, religion, or sexual orientation."[30] Physicians and their patients react to the quality of their exchange, potentially withdrawing from uncomfortable and unpleasant interactions. Physicians' responses to patients can influence their behavior, serving as a means of social control. In repeated interactions, patients learn what behaviors are rewarded or appreciated and what behaviors might result in abrupt interactions and limited communication. Judith Lorber has found that surgical inpatients who disrupted normative routines were labeled "problem patients" by physicians and floor nurses and that consequences of this label included premature discharge, neglect, and referral to a psychiatrist.[31]

Medical practitioners are not immune to being punished by patients or by patients' family members. Workplace violence remains a challenge for medical staff, especially for nurses and emergency room physicians. The World Health Organization estimates that globally, 8%–38% of healthcare workers will experience physical violence at some point during their career.[32] One study in Minnesota found that 13% of nurses experienced physical assault per year, while 39% experienced threats, sexual harassment, and verbal abuse per year.[33] About 50% of emergency room physicians have been assaulted, a risk they attribute in part to working with a patient population who suffers from mental health issues, drug abuse, and stress from understaffed departments.[34] The risk of experiencing workplace violence tragically increased during the COVID-19 pandemic.[35,36]

In the absence of mental health challenges and drug abuse, why might patients still abuse members of their medical team? Given the extreme stress from experiencing a potentially significant illness episode, and considering patients' vulnerable state, cast into an unfamiliar and complex medical institution, they might lash out as an expression of their fear and desperation, much like a cornered animal. While we might conceptually understand the impetus for the abusive behavior, the consequence for the patient may be dire if their behavior causes their medical team to withdraw from providing the best care and communicating effectively with the patient.

My Attempts to Be a Good Patient

I started feeling overwhelmed by the demands of numerous medical appointments early in my cancer experience. I began to recognize interaction fatigue during the months of tests and procedures leading up to my eventual diagnosis. Human beings are simultaneously highly social animals who also require regular and meaningful breaks from social interactions. Erving Goffman again provides a framework in his *Presentation of Self in Everyday Life* for thinking of these two essential selves as our "front-stage" and "backstage" identities.[37] Our front-stage lives are enacted in numerous public institutional settings—from our office spaces, to the grocery store, to the concerts we attend. We are performing our social roles in front of others, and during these encounters, Goffman argues, we try to control people's impression of us through our words and actions. Feeling as though we are succeeding in this impression management satisfies our social identities. In our backstage lives, we are released from the stress and pressure of continually trying to control numerous others' impressions of us. Others may be with us in our backstage settings, such as family members or roommates in our homes, but these social scripts are less rigid, and ideally, acceptance and support are part of our backstage relationships.

Many of us find it hard to interact with people every day, whether these people are our colleagues in the workplace or the clients we serve, even if we have good, collegial relationships and perhaps count these people among our friends. Even during our most intimate interactions in the backstages of our lives, following the rules of productive and healthy interactions for hours at a time is hard—maintain eye contact, smile (or at least avoid scowling), be attentive, be kind, take turns, be respectful, and so forth. As much as I love teaching, there are times when I just do not feel like walking into the classroom, or seeing students during my office hours, or interacting with my colleagues in the hallway or at a meeting. Sociologists who study workplace settings talk about the ways office organization reveals information about relationships between workers and power structures.[38] Consider the luxury of having a private office (and not just a cubicle) where someone can retreat, even if only for a while, from the demands of social work lives. Line-level workers often function in public institutional spaces under the watchful eye of management, while members of management are rewarded with offices with doors that they can close.

During the diagnostic stage of my cancer experience, and shortly into the treatment stage, I became very aware of the challenges of interacting with medical professionals and staff members so often. I sometimes found it extremely challenging to be "nice," perky, pleasant, and so forth with so many different people, especially when I was feeling so poorly, and because they were often poking and prodding me, scanning my body parts, and/or injecting me with antibodies and chemotherapy drugs. And yet I was also very aware of how much I wanted my entire treatment team—from the clerical staff, to the phlebotomists, to the oncology nurses, to my oncologist—to like me.

People who know me well know that I am not someone who spends much time concerned about whether people "like" me. I am very aware that I am not everyone's "cup of tea," and I know that "you can't please everyone all the time." While as a sociologist, I am absolutely fascinated with people and the human experience in general, and therefore professionally tolerant of the full spectrum of human behavior, personally, I am demanding of others. I expect people to be kind and fair, use their talents, fulfill their obligations, and think beyond the confines of their own life experiences—standards that serve me well as a university sociology professor but that do not necessarily make me an easy person with whom to interact.

While I am not concerned about being "likeable," I do find that people tend to find me "approachable." How do I know this? Here is an example: Almost every time I go to the supermarket, a stranger interacts with me. I often am asked my opinion about a product or what I am planning to make for dinner. The people interacting with me reflect a wide range of demographic characteristics—young and old, displaying male or female, varying races, and so forth. I suspect that people talk to me because I tend to smile when I am in public. I smile as a part of my own socialization as a female (I have yet to meet someone above age fourteen who identifies or who gets identified as a female and has not been told to smile in public)—smiling is part of my front-stage performance. But I also smile because I generally enjoy being out and about in public. For example, I actually like to shop for groceries, so I do smile in the supermarket. I also tend to smile the entire time I am walking my dogs or walking around a nature preserve. I do tend to enjoy life and enjoy life's various activities. I also greatly enjoy people-watching, and so I tend to make eye contact with strangers wherever I go. I suspect that the act of making eye contact while smiling is interpreted as an invitation to interact with me.

I have basically described myself as someone who is demanding but at least initially approachable, but during my treatment, I wanted to be more than that when I was functioning as a patient. I wanted to be likeable, *really* likeable. I was acutely aware of my desire to have my physicians, nurses, and all the staff members like me. And the chasm between my desire to be likeable and my at-times-perceived shortcomings to be such, especially when I was feeling very poorly or was very depressed, was concerning.

Why was I suddenly so concerned about being likeable? Having professionally studied medical practitioners for my entire career, I have the utmost respect for people who choose the healing professions. I have studied intently their socialization process, the demands of their professional training, and I admire and applaud their commitment, their values, and their vocational calling to do this kind of work. I have so much admiration for medical practitioners as a general occupational category that I want them to respect and admire me in return. This desire is not easy in the current configuration of the delivery of medical care. I have also studied physician burnout and know that everyone working in the profession believes that there are too many patients and not enough time to provide the best comprehensive care for everyone.[39] Knowing that my time with each professional was short and jam-packed with information that needed to be covered and shared made it even more imperative that I was in top form myself—recall the good patient script discussed earlier: Maintain eye contact, smile, listen carefully, ask good questions, use this time well, and make a really good joke if you can so that they will remember you! Be likeable! Be the patient whom they might talk about over dinner later that day with their family members. "I had the nicest appointment today with one of my patients. . . ."

Therefore, I was in part driven by my desire to be liked by people whom I admire, but I also had another motivation: I wanted to be liked because I wanted these people to take the very best care of me that they could. I understood that my life was on the line, that my life was literally in their hands, and I wanted to make sure that everyone who was involved in my treatment cared about whether I survived. I know that these professionals are driven by their own ethics to treat *all* of their patients equally and provide the best care to everyone, but from my perspective, I thought, if this professional feels comfortable with me, likes me, will they not be in the best state of mind to make sure that all my tests are correct, all my medications are correct, and my doses are appropriate? Should I have a poor reaction, will they not be more inclined to come just as fast as they possibly can to my rescue? So, in retrospect, being very "likeable" was part of my overall attempt to do everything possible to increase my likelihood of surviving. Since studies have shown that at least 15% of patients are deemed "difficult" by the medical practitioners treating them, with some more recent studies putting that number closer to 30%, I clearly wanted to be in the 70%–85% "not difficult" category.[40] And ideally, because I am also a bit competitive, I really wanted to be on my practitioners' lists of "favorite" patients!

Later, in Chapter 10, I share some stories about some of the problematic patient behavior I witnessed.

The Terrible, Horrible, No Good, Very Bad War Metaphors Used to Describe the Cancer Experience

Our medical language is full of war imagery. Illness and death are the ultimate enemies! We must fight the invaders! We will pull out all the "big guns" to battle illness! As part of our sick role, we must do everything possible to overcome illness and delay death. We must, as Dylan Thomas tells us, "Rage, rage against the dying of the light."[1]

Some of the ills we experience are indeed caused by invaders—parasites, viruses, bacteria. These are foreign organisms (enemies, if you will) that may break through our defenses and wreak havoc on our bodies. They may threaten our health (and, at times, our very lives), our ability to fully function, and we need to rid ourselves of these intruders, either through our own immune responses or with a little help from medical interventions, to be restored to full health and functioning. Susan Sontag tells us that the first wide use of war metaphors—the enemy and the battle—to describe illness and our attempts to restore health surfaced in the 1880s, with the identification of bacteria as causes of disease.[2]

But the extensive use of war metaphors in healthcare, and the suggestion that all foreign substances—all bacteria, for example—are deleterious, has not necessarily had a positive impact on our approach to managing our health, on our attempts to live in harmony with other organisms in our environment, and even on our treatment of disease. For example, the well-documented rise over the past few decades in the development of asthma and allergies among children growing up in modern industrialized nations has been linked to lack of exposure to diverse environmental microbes.[3] In short, immune systems developing in overly sterile environments do not develop properly—this observation has been termed the *hygiene hypothesis*.[4,5,6] Evidence even suggests that babies born via C-section, who are denied the benefit of being exposed to beneficial intestinal microbes during a vaginal delivery, are at greater risk of developing allergy disorders, so this negative impact can begin at birth.[7] A poorly developed immune system has also been linked to the development of autoimmune disorders.[8]

Sanitation is very important to maintaining human health and increasing life expectancy, but the trick is finding the balance between enough exposure to germs to help the immune system develop and overexposure, which can overwhelm the system and cause permanent damage or death. Extensive debates about how we achieve this balance grew as we negotiated and tried to identify appropriate levels of exposure to endemic pathogens during a pandemic.

Evidence of soap use in human communities has been found as early as 2800 B.C.E. in Babylonia. Bathing was also common among the residents of Rome in the sixth century B.C.E., and the expansion of the Roman Empire brought Rome's soapmaking techniques and bathing habits to conquered lands in Europe, but with the fall of the Roman Empire in A.D. 467, Europeans abandoned many of their bathing habits, contributing to the highly unsanitary conditions of the Middle Ages.[9] Residents in Italy, Spain, and France did continue soap manufacturing, in part due to their ready supply of source materials, such as olive oil. But it was not until the seventeenth century that bathing and soap use came back into fashion in much of Europe. Demographers postulate that increased personal and public health sanitation measures, along with increased nutrition, significantly reduced mortality rates in Europe in the eighteenth century.[10,11]

As suggested in the previous paragraph, the product traditionally called "soap" is made from fats or oils, and any source of fat—animal or vegetable. Fat is transformed into soap when mixed with an alkali.[12] Most of the products we use today for cleaning are not soaps by this definition but chemical detergents. The switch from soaps to detergents was driven by fat shortages experienced during WWI and WWII. Chemists used other available raw materials to produce solutions with similar cleaning properties to those of traditional soap.[9]

After WWII, we saw an increased focus on the importance of housekeeping in American society and the desire to create sterile environments. The impetuses for this greater focus were multiple. One was the changing role of women in society. During the war, many women, some of whom had worked as maids before the war, entered the formal wage labor market to fill vital production roles left vacant by the male soldiers who went off to fight in Europe. The period from 1940–1945 saw the largest growth in female participation in the formal labor force during the entire twentieth century, growing from 28% to 34%.[13] Once the war ended, many of these women were forced out of the labor market to make room for the returning men. But many of the women who had been maids did not want to return to this work, leaving American households without an adequate supply of maid labor to meet the demand, and so we entered the era of the "housewife."[14] This higher standard of the clean home was also driven by the producers of the new cleaning detergents created during the wars, which needed a market for their products. The housewife became the target consumer, and the home environment the applied site. By 1965, despite advances in detergents and in technology, such as electric cleaning appliances (for example, the vacuum cleaner), that should have made housekeeping easier, the standard of what constituted an adequately clean home was so demanding that women were spending more time on housekeeping tasks—an average of fifty-five hours per week—than their grandmothers had.[15] We adopted war metaphors to describe our housework, referring to "fighting" and "winning the war" against germs and doing "battle against" dust.[16,17]

When we adopt the view that germs are the enemy that must be destroyed/eliminated, how do we know how much exposure is appropriate for the development and maintenance of our immune systems? When should we not rush to wash and sterilize the child's pacifier? How sterile should our home environments be? How often should we wash our hands? How often should we get at least a bit sick, when we are young and as we grow older, so that our immune systems continue to remember how to function appropriately, avoiding a hyper- or insufficient immune response?

The War Metaphor and Our Views about Cancer

Cancer is the disease that Americans fear the most, and it tops the list of Americans' greatest overall fears.[18] This fear is fed in part by the way mass media primarily portrays cancer—as something to be feared, almost inevitable—while highlighting the scariest statistics.[19] As Sontag argues, cancer has been so feared throughout human history that it has become core to our political lexicon. Threats to social order are often referred to as "cancers" by those in power, and this label invites strong action against whatever threat is identified, be it changes in social norms, growing migrant populations, challenges to power structures, and so forth. Referring to events as cancers taps into, maintains, and reinforces our general fears.[2] Studies have shown that people view cancer as "a vicious, unpredictable, and indestructible enemy, evoking fears about its proximity, the (lack of) strategies to keep it at bay, the personal and social implications of succumbing, and fear of dying from cancer."[20]

Some have theorized that presenting cancer through war imagery helps mobilize people to pay attention to their bodies and seek screening opportunities since the earlier in the stage of development that the cancer is discovered, the better the prognosis. But studies have suggested that battle metaphors increase fatalistic beliefs and may lead patients to delay seeking medical attention.[21]

How has the medical war metaphor influenced our approach to treating cancer? Think of the warlike terms we often associate with all types of cancers—cancer is described as aggressive, malignant, invasive, destructive, and so forth. These terms are not surprising, given how cancer was experienced and described throughout human history prior to any forms of effective treatment. War terminology is also not surprising since the first chemotherapy drugs came about as a result of discoveries made during WWII:

> During World War II, naval personnel who were exposed to mustard gas during military action were found to have toxic changes in the bone marrow cells that develop into blood cells. During that same period, the US Army was studying a number of chemicals related to mustard gas to develop more effective agents for war and also develop protective measures. In the course of that work, a compound called nitrogen mustard was studied and found to work against a cancer of the lymph nodes called lymphoma. . . . Not long after the discovery of nitrogen mustard, Sidney Farber of Boston demonstrated that aminopterin, a compound related to the vitamin folic acid, produced remissions in children with acute leukemia. Aminopterin blocked a critical chemical reaction needed for DNA replication. That drug was the predecessor of methotrexate, a cancer treatment drug used commonly today. Since then, other researchers discovered drugs that block different functions in cell growth and replication. The era of chemo-

therapy had begun. Metastatic cancer was first cured in 1956 when methotrexate was used to treat a rare tumor called choriocarcinoma.[22]

Once we finally had some ways to battle cancer, early treatment protocols were typically very aggressive, in part influenced by our fear of the disease and our desire to conquer this enemy, and in part due to the theory that cancer could be conquered only through total destruction.[23] In due course, physicians recalibrated some of the original protocols since they realized that while they were destroying cancer cells, they were also destroying too many of their patients' healthy cells by administering more chemotherapy and radiation than was necessary to achieve remission, in some cases causing permanent disability and significantly raising risks for secondary cancers caused by the treatments. Continuing modifications in dosages have resulted in better "cocktails," more refined surgical procedures, and better treatment schedules. Less-aggressive treatment was often better. Consider, for example, the significantly increased use of lumpectomies instead of total mastectomies for the management of breast cancer.[24]

Cancer as the Enemy

While we modify how aggressively we manage cancer treatments, cancer is still talked about as an "enemy" against which the patient is "battling."[25,26] But here is where the war metaphor about fighting an invader fails: Cancer is not a foreign organism that has invaded the patient's body. Cancer cells are the patient's cells gone rogue. While the cancer might have been triggered by an outside agent, virus, substance, and so forth, those "carcinogens" are not necessarily still present in the patient's body. So, if you say that the patient is battling cancer, the patient is, in essence, battling themselves. I have met the enemy, and it is me? What does the cancer patient do with this realization? How might my relationship with my body change, knowing that some part of me seriously malfunctioned? Do I feel betrayed by myself? Do I start to do battle with myself? And if you set me up for a battle, how do I interpret the patients whose treatments do not work, who eventually die? Did they not fight hard enough? And what about those who face high risk of recurrence, whose battle might not end soon, or ever?[27] How might the battle imagery be damaging and burdensome for the illness narratives all cancer patients are trying to compose? If patients are required to constantly battle and forge ahead, do we remove any opportunity for them to express their fear and to mourn the diagnosis?[28]

My Complicated and Ever-Changing
Relationship with My Body

Many people in Western Christian cultures hold to some degree the view that the mind and body are distinct and separate, a view also known as mind-body dualism, a view credited to René Descartes in the seventeenth century.[29] Who I am is essentially defined by my thoughts, my consciousness, and who I essentially "am" cannot be lessened by some biological explanation, reducible to some causal explanation of brain cells firing. I am greater than the sum of my cells, greater than my biology. Many people who hold this view also give greater precedence to the mind. The mind is the master, and the body is the vehicle (temple) for the mind. And the field of modern medicine has been driven to a significant degree by this dualism, reducing the study and understanding of the body to its various components and not viewing health in relation to the entire functioning body living in a community and in an environment.[30]

Since my diagnosis, I have often thought about my own views about the mind-body dualism. When we are no longer healthy, we are bitterly and brutally reminded that the dualism is false. My mind and body are wholly linked. I cannot abuse my body. After my lymphoma diagnosis, I was reminded that my mind, my essence, my very existence was contingent on restoring my body to a state of health.

Illness reminds us that the master—the power of our minds—has some serious limitations. I could not consciously "think" myself well. All my conscious deliberations, musings, considerations, and so forth, all the power of my rational cognitive functioning could not command my rogue "large B cells" back into proper functioning. And my cancer diagnosis also led me to reflect on my long relationship with my body.

Like most women growing up in America, I had deeply internalized the messages in my childhood and adolescence that I was not quite enough—not pretty enough, not thin enough, not athletic enough, not smooth enough, too small in the chest, too big in the thigh. And I, too, felt that using products and modifying behaviors were my responsibility. Apply the numerous creams and lotions; eat the cottage cheese diet, the grapefruit diet, count the calories; ride the bike, jog, do aerobics. The mind was master and most important, but a particular kind of body was also highly valued, a social asset, and expected. During these formative years, I cannot say that I had a very good relationship with my body. It seemed to continually let me down, no matter how hard I tried to meet the standards.

In college, I fell in love with the field of sociology, and once I recognized that beauty is a social construct, I began to throw off the yoke of a particular, limited, burdensome definition of what constitutes a good body and started developing a new relationship with it. Nurturing this new relationship was not easy, and for a very long time, I would feel the pangs associated with not measuring up to some contrived ideal, for these early internalized expectations run very deep, and the idealized body is marketed to us on a daily basis, so it is hard to ignore. This marketing is designed to make us continue to buy the creams, eat the special diets, use the special exercise equipment. The beauty industry flourished when it successfully convinced us that we are not enough and are not doing enough.

But for many years, I dwelled happily in my body. My mind and body came to a wonderful arrangement: I would take care of it, using all the knowledge at my disposal of how to keep it healthy (especially eating well and getting regular exercise), I would not abuse it too much, and in return, my body would allow me to fulfill the roles and partake in the activities in my life that bring me great joy, that help define who I am, and that allow me to interact with others, to laugh, to stand in awe before nature, to engage with others. And until February 2019, my mind and body fully enjoyed cooking, drawing, gardening, golfing, laughing, taking long walks/hikes, parenting, experiencing romance, singing, shopping (farmers markets and arts and crafts, primarily), playing soccer and squash, socializing, swimming in the ocean, teaching, and writing. But then my body let me know that everything was not okay and that I had to give up some of these cherished activities. And with each activity that I lost through the process of diagnosis and treatment, I also lost a sense of myself, a source of joy, a source of meaning in my life. During the course of my diagnosis and treatment, I transitioned from being "Ginny" to being what often felt like a full-time patient.

What was my relationship with my body during treatment? I was terribly disappointed. I caught myself sometimes looking at my right humerus, shaking my head. How could you betray me like that? But I also acknowledged that my humerus (and my other cancer sites) were not my enemy, were not foreign invaders. They were and are me. Since the enemy analogy did not work well in this case, what other ways of envisioning this process helped me navigate the very complex emotions I felt and continue to feel? A biological process went awry, and I worked to get all my systems back on track. The process was a reboot, a reset—a rebirth, if you will.

I experienced significant overlap between how I felt during chemotherapy and how I felt when I was pregnant—nauseated, very fatigued, craving protein and vinegar. And I found myself taking comfort in this familiarity. I consumed poisons that killed off the malfunctioning parts of myself so that they could be supplanted by properly functioning replacements—that part of me was reborn. The notion that from the wreckage left behind by these chemotherapeutic agents, new life arose, new cells were born, inspired hope. It also inspired me to have compassionate thoughts about my own body, about all the work it did. And I was a little less frustrated, a little less disappointed. I was not in battle with myself. I was in the process of a rebirth. For my next tattoo (I already had a rose and a sunflower), I got a phoenix on my right upper arm, right over my humerus. The pandemic delayed this acquisition, but it eventually happened.

Is there a better way to envision and describe the cancer patient's experience? Some researchers are calling for an increased use of the term *journey* and related metaphors as more meaningful, cross-culturally appropriate alternatives to military metaphors. Later, in Chapter 12, I review some positive and negative functions of using journey metaphors to describe the cancer experience.

The Challenges of Interacting with Family, Friends, Neighbors, and Acquaintances and Responding to "How Are You?"

Recall from Chapter 4 our discussion of Erving Goffman's presentation of self and front-stage performance and of Charles Horton Cooley's looking-glass self as we explored the transformation of the individual into a cancer patient. The often-extensive physical changes that result from treatment and the accompanying extreme fatigue demand that patients adapt to new ways of presenting self and affect their communication strategies with medical personnel. All these changes also significantly influence patients' communication styles with family, friends, neighbors, and the numerous strangers we encounter every day. They also influence the types of communications we have in medical settings versus those we have in other institutional settings.

Let us first consider the normal exchanges we have with strangers in common daily settings. Numerous times a day in modern society, we interact with strangers at the grocery store, the post office, while driving, or even with "strangers" at our workplaces, people we might recognize by sight but with whom we have not exchanged even minor pleasantries. In every interaction, no matter how brief, we follow internalized rules of behavior to manage our self-presentation during these encounters, adjusting our behavior as we imagine how we are being seen and experienced by the other to achieve a successful interaction. Successful interactions typically share these most basic factors—we demonstrate good intentions, we maintain social harmony, and we successfully complete the transaction.[1]

When at the grocery store, as we are about to check out, the employee working at the register will often ask "How are you?," and the vast majority of us respond, "Good, how are you?" Once this exchange happens, we commence our interaction. The employee scans my goods, I pay for my groceries, and we often share a quick "good-bye" at the end, with perhaps an added "Have a nice day!" Even though a close reading of the employee's original question suggests that they are asking us to share information about our state of being (How am I? My physical state? My emotional state?), we know that we are not expected to share any details about how we are, nor do we think that the person asking actually wants to know these details.

The purpose of the question "How are you?" is to see whether you are ready for a social interaction with one of the many "strangers" whom we encounter every single day in modern societies. It is a social convention. Very few of us ever actually respond to the supermarket employee with some "honest" detailed commentary on "how we are" at that moment.

To illustrate the meaning behind these ritualized exchanges for students in my introductory sociology class, I ask them to violate the norm in an exchange with someone in a common social interaction, such as with the person checking them out at the supermarket: When the person asks how they are, respond with something negative, something other than "okay," to see how the questioner reacts. For most of my life, I have experienced migraine headaches, and when I have a migraine, I occasionally tell the stranger asking me how I am that I currently have one. Responding with "I have a migraine" typically throws off the supermarket employee, and they usually take a few seconds to respond. What I find fascinating is that a common response is often an attempt to reestablish the connection that was interrupted by my unexpected reply. One of the most typical is to share with me their own headache experiences or to tell me about someone they know who gets migraines. Once our connection is restored, we continue our interaction. At the end of the transaction, instead of saying, "Have a nice day," they usually say, "Feel better soon!" Most people quickly adjust, even when the norm is violated.

Deviating even briefly from deeply internalized normative behaviors can get us to think about the function they serve and what those expected exchanges communicate about our relationships with others in our society. The question "How are you?" and the answers we might give vary greatly, depending on whether that person is a stranger, a friend, a family member, and so forth. It might be the exact same question, but it has incredibly different weight, interpretation, and acceptable responses. These differences illustrate

Goffman's distinction between our front-stage and backstage performances. We are more "honest" with the people we invite backstage. We do not have to be as careful to craft their impressions of us. We share the backstage with our intimates, who are defined by our ability to be our authentic selves in their presence. When an intimate asks how we are, we can ideally lose the façade of surface social harmony and functioning and share our lived reality.

Being Asked "How Are You?" in Medical Settings

It is somewhat odd that personnel in medical offices often employ the same social conventions as the supermarket employee or the waitstaff at a restaurant to establish the first connection, given how different our experiences are in a medical setting versus other institutions. The nurse walking you back to the exam room might casually ask, "How are you today?" Patients are aware that the nurse is not literally asking you to start giving details about your physical or emotional state at that moment—the question functions as the initial small-talk exchange. But I have often been tempted to respond, "I am not well. In fact, I'm pretty upset, as I am here seeing you as an emergency visit" or "I am sick enough that I made an appointment. I am in a great deal of pain and would frankly rather be anywhere other than here." Despite this temptation, most of us complete the expected script, perhaps adding a statement or two about the weather, and then once we're in the exam room, we try to honestly communicate how we are feeling. If I am going to a medical appointment for anything other than a well visit, it is likely that I am not okay.

I reflected on the dysfunctional aspect of these types of questions in medical settings as I sought an explanation for the severe pain in my right arm. After my insurance company denied my physician's requests for a PET scan, as noted in Chapter 1, it finally agreed to a bone biopsy since a bone scan showed "activity" in my right humerus. When I was getting prepped for the procedure, two nurses were elevating me in a way that made my humerus most accessible for the biopsy, getting me hooked up to monitors and prepped for the anesthesiologist. Both of them were wonderfully kind and informative. They explained everything that they were doing and the reasons for particular manipulations. But as all this activity was happening to and around me, I was overwhelmed by the reality of what was about to happen (they are going to drill into my bone and withdraw a sample of my marrow!), and I started to shed some tears. One of the nurses immediately came over and asked me, "What's wrong?," and I remember thinking, "Isn't it obvious what is wrong?"

I looked back at his very kind face and said, "I'm about to have a bone bi-opsy." He laughed a genuine, lovely laugh, squeezed my hand, and told me that they would take care of me. But this exchange made me wonder, don't most patients about to undergo a surgical procedure cry, even a little bit? Was I breaking an expected code of behavior? Was I failing to be stoic enough? If every person about to undergo a procedure had a significant breakdown, this reaction would certainly interfere with the functioning of the institution, but aren't some expressions of fear and grief to be expected? I took comfort in the fact that I had made the nurse laugh, and I believed that they would take care of me. As I was coming out of the anesthesia from this procedure, the young surgeon (she looked *so* young to me that day) was proudly telling the team about the quality of the samples she had drawn from my bone. I doubt that she knew that I could hear her, and while I was happy that the procedure appeared to be successful, I was still terrified at that moment of what the samples might reveal.

Another example occurred at the office of an oral surgeon. During treat-ment, I developed a terrible toothache. The tooth was beyond repair and had to be pulled—not an easy procedure to schedule while I was already deep into treatment and immunocompromised. I had an emergency appointment with an oral surgeon, and when I arrived at this office and was being taken back to the exam room, the nurse started making small talk, asking me whether I was "having a nice summer." I looked at her incredulously. Here I was, bald, without eyelashes and only minimal eyebrows, and in extensive pain from the toothache, and she was asking whether I was having a nice summer. I re-sponded honestly, clearly violating the expected exchange. I told her that I was having a horrible summer since I was spending it as a cancer patient! In this case, we could have made small talk about the weather, nonpolitical current events, or the performance of regional sports teams, avoiding questions that might potentially lead to deep existential grief. No, I am not having a nice summer, I am trying to stay alive.

Although I experienced her question as a misreading of her audience, I did understand that she did not normally deal with cancer patients with emer-gency tooth issues in this particular private practice office. Conversely, at the Perelman Center at the University of Pennsylvania, the substantial multistory healthcare facility where I saw my oncologist and got my outpatient infusions, you cannot stand in the atrium, take an elevator ride, or look at the people all around you without acknowledging that the vast majority of those people are not at all "good, fine, well" and that they would rather be a hundred—no, a thousand—other places than there. It is devastatingly poignant. So many cancer patients and their families and friends pass through that building every day that Penn has hired special staff members whose job it is to help people find spaces in the parking lot, work the elevators, find their physician's office. I noticed that these special concierges never asked me, "How are you?" when beginning our interaction. They instead asked, "Do you need any assistance? Do you need directions? Do you need help finding . . . ?" And I wondered and continue to wonder whether they had been instructed explicitly not to ask, "How are you?," as perhaps we can all acknowledge that in this setting, the answer is often fraught and extremely complicated. And perhaps it is easier for us as we are getting ready to see the doctor, have the scan, get the biopsy, receive the infusion not to focus on "how we are" but rather to accept the kindness of the person who can facilitate our journey to where we need to be. Do you need assistance? Yes, that would be lovely, thank you.

Running Into a Friend on the Street

As noted in Chapter 7, cancer is the most feared disease in American society. And for many cancer patients, it is not easy to hide the side effects from treatment, even if they want to. Given the underlying fear of cancer that so many people have, it is not hard to understand how this fear might lead to their attempt to downplay the severity of the experience, if they are willing to acknowledge it in the first place, when interacting with the patient. Engaging in normative banter on the sidewalk or in the local market is significantly challenged and informed by the level of relationship, by the degree to which the person is or is not an intimate. Depending on how the exchange unfolds and how successfully both parties experience the exchange, relationships may get redefined, for better or for worse.

As noted earlier, during my months of treatment, I tried to make sure that I walked at least a couple of miles every day, as I was aware of the correlation between exercise and successful treatment. Since about half of my treatment occurred during the summer, I was often out and about on sunny summer afternoons and ended up running into many friends also on walks or running errands in our little town center. Before being diagnosed with lymphoma, I regularly interacted with many local friends while playing soccer and squash. During treatment, I did not play either of these sports, but most people learned through various communication routes that I had cancer.

Because of photosensitivity from treatment, when I went for a walk or ran errands, I typically wore my favorite baseball cap. Other times, I wore a large sun-protection hat, so it was not always immediately obvious when looking at me that I had lost my hair. When running into a friend I knew from many hours on the soccer field or squash court during this time, quickly following the expected, "How are you?," I would be quite frank about my current situation. I would tell them that the treatments were brutal, that the fatigue was indescribable, that the whole process was terrifying. And often by their response, I would realize that I had been a bit too honest. Wearing an uncomfortable expression, they most commonly responded to my honesty with "Well, you *look* great!"

My reaction to being told that I looked great was complicated. While I am confident that friends said this in part to reduce my suffering, to inject a bit of positivity, it also had the effect of ending an honest discussion of the experience—it served their desire to cut short the narrative and to avoid an unhappy topic. It also bizarrely seemed to question the validity of my perspective—could it really be that bad if I still looked as good as I did? Did my outward appearance right now not adequately reflect the chaos and damage that was occurring on a cellular level inside my body? Should I have carried around my blood work results and scans to prove the trauma? The response was also problematic as typically the person did not first acknowledge the struggles I had just described. A friend dealing with ovarian cancer said to me that she often avoided wearing makeup because its presence made people assume that she was okay and feeling fine.

Having some friends dodge the discussion or disregard my narrative did end up affecting some relationships. People who had been in my inner circles stepped out, and that felt harsh. People with whom I had shared happy and challenging personal stories about such vitally central life issues as child-rearing, marriage, and work seemed unwilling, but perhaps really unable, to hear some of the most challenging stories in my life. My life, at least during treatment, was a bit too tragic. Some friends morphed into acquaintances.

Ghosting Is Common

A recent informal survey of cancer patients found that 65% reported being ghosted by people in their lives after their cancer diagnosis—people withdrew without explanation.[2] Part of the withdrawal may be explained by our deep fear of the disease. While cancer is not contagious in the common ways we think of contagion, people might be afraid that sharing a newly diagnosed individual's "environment" could increase their own chance of developing cancer.

Another factor contributing to ghosting might stem from our ultra-optimism, a core cultural trait of American society since its founding. Alexis de Tocqueville, a French diplomat, famously observed this optimism during a trip to the United States in the early nineteenth century, and he highlights this climate of extreme American optimism in his book *Democracy in America*.[3] And this American optimism has continued. In a 2015 survey by the Pew Research Center, Americans expressed their belief that they have control over their lives and that hard work pays off, and they reported at the time of the survey having a "particularly good day."[4] Part of Americans' national identity is to "look on the bright side" of life.[5] Being pessimistic, sharing bad news, and taking off the rose-colored glasses are not tolerated, especially in the public domain. Responding to someone's tragic illness narrative with "You look good!" may be an attempt to meet the normative demands of public banter.

But another explanation might be that we do not know how to maintain relationships with people who might die. Despite recent advances in remission rates for many cancers, Americans still believe that cancer is a death sentence.[6] As noted by Myra Bluebond-Langner, author of *The Private Worlds of Dying Children*, we are challenged to maintain normal relationships with people we fear might die.[7] Normal relationships, which are often informed by references to the future, are tested by the possibility of death. Why spend time and share meals, social acts that serve as investments in a friendship, with a person who might no longer be around in a few months? Why would the ill individual facing mortality continue to participate in the activities that maintain their membership in a community? For the cancer patient in treatment to continue, there must be hope of reassuming their membership.

In public, the cancer patient could don an "everything is okay" façade. This performance could actually be rewarded if the façade keeps others comfortable and limits ghosting. The patient could be the "brave warrior," admired by friends and neighbors. Speaking truth to the trauma threatens the social order. But is the façade functional for the patient?

Acknowledging the Trauma

Cancer patients experience trauma throughout their illness experience, and as for other groups who experience trauma—"war veterans, children, and people who have been through a physical or sexual assault, abuse, accident, disaster,

or other serious events"—treatment can help manage the dysfunctional impacts of the trauma experience on everyday life.[8] The development of post-
traumatic stress disorder (PTSD) is more common than we might expect. On
the whole, about seven or eight out of every hundred people will experience
PTSD at some point in their lives, with about one-third of people being exposed to a significant trauma event.[9]

Studies show that PTSD remains underdiagnosed and, therefore, under-
treated, even within mental health settings. In a study conducted by Drew
Miele and Edward J. O'Brien, the published rate of diagnosis of PTSD in
mental health programs for children and adolescents in Pennsylvania was 2%
and 5%, respectively. The researchers did their own standardized diagnostic
review and found that the rates were actually 48% and 45%, respectively, at
the two sites. Licensed mental health clinicians were missing the diagnosis of
PTSD.[10,11]

Physicians increasingly acknowledge that a consequence of modern medical treatment for the seriously ill may be PTSD. A study conducted by a team
of investigators at the Johns Hopkins University School of Medicine found
that one-fifth of critically ill patients who had been in intensive care had
PTSD symptoms even one-year posttreatment.[12,13]

And PTSD is well documented among cancer patients. The rates of PTSD
vary somewhat by the site of the cancer (breast versus bone, for example) and
the point of measurement (shortly after diagnosis or posttreatment), ranging
from about 7%–53%, but are consistently higher than in the general population. And all the studies call for better screening and treatment methods for
cancer patients with PTSD.[14,15,16]

Since the normative rules of social interaction significantly limit patients'
ability to discuss their trauma with only their closest intimates, even though
the trauma is well documented and prevalent, as I discuss in subsequent chapters, support groups become vital communities. As I have noted in previous
chapters, patients are understandably reluctant to voice their trauma to the
members of their medical teams for fear of being viewed as problematic and
ungrateful, or for fear of reminding the professionals themselves of their own
limitations to "do no harm." But the support group can become a front-stage
setting where patients can talk about their trauma, receive unquestionably
empathetic support, and have their stories told, honored, and shared. The
cancer patient is freed from the backstage, behind the curtain, corners. But it
would also be incredibly helpful if our friends and neighbors could sit with us,
even briefly, with the honest challenges we face during treatment.

Touch and Treatment

Touch is the most fundamental of our senses.[1] Consider that it is through touch that human beings first experience and explore their world. Studies show that babies deprived of human touch have delayed development and that these delays may negatively affect them throughout their lives.[2,3] All the specific mechanisms through which touch aids cognitive development are still under investigation, but it has been established that touch decreases stress hormones, such as cortisol, and increases beneficial bonding hormones, such as oxytocin.[4] These hormonal impacts affect the function of our immune systems.

And touch remains an important component of our physical and emotional well-being throughout our lives. The need for touch may increase later in life as hearing and vision become increasingly impaired. In particular, elderly impaired individuals may need touch to communicate and remain connected to people.[5,6]

But touch can also be fraught throughout our lifetime and differ by cultural settings. Each society has rules about who has permission to touch our bodies, where they can touch, to whom we bestow hugs and kisses, and these rules change based on our age and the state of our relationship, especially as we enter different sexual and reproductive stages of our lives. Sandra J. Weiss, a cardiologist, has identified six tactile symbols that influence how touch is experienced: duration, location, action, intensity, frequency, and sensation.[7] The appropriateness of a touch is assessed by the successful meeting of these symbols, and specific rules apply in different medical settings regarding what constitutes required and acceptable touches. The kinds of touches expected when seeing an otolaryngologist are significantly different than those expected when seeing a gynecologist, for example.

In the case of cancer, the unfounded fear of contagion and people's general significant fear of the "disease" can render the cancer patient even more "touch-hungry" than other patients since others in their lives may have significantly decreased how often they touch the cancer patient post diagnosis.[8] This unmet need for touch may make caring and comforting touches even more vital during oncology appointments.

Touch as Introduction

A common way for people to greet each other in Western societies is to shake hands. The COVID-19 pandemic interrupted this ritual since we recognized that our hands are some of the most germ-coated parts of our bodies and that we consistently pass viruses and bacteria to each other via our hands. We have experimented with fist bumps or elbow shakes, but with its long history, the handshake will likely stay with us.[9,10] Handshaking is a deeply embedded ritualized behavior that carries rich and varying meanings in different institutional settings, from the family gathering, to the religious ceremony (think of the reception line at a wedding), to work settings where deals are made.

The history of the handshake dates back almost three thousand years, when it was depicted on ancient Greek reliefs and gravestones.[11] Handshaking is believed by historians to have begun as a way to show another that you were not holding any weapons, which is why the right hand is most often used. Shaking was a way to show that there were no hidden weapons up your sleeve. Bjarke Oxlund, an anthropologist, has also reviewed the transition from this early meaning to the handshake as a way to make and seal deals, to the use by Quakers as a sign of equality between people, a deliberate rejection of bowing and curtsying.[3]

Deborah Schiffrin, a sociolinguist, categorizes the handshake into three main types: openers, closures, and collapses.[12] The first describes the handshake that establishes interaction between two actors. The second type concludes an agreed-upon period of interaction, and the third combines both, serving simultaneously as a greeting and a farewell, such as the handshake we share with a passing politician or celebrity.

Studies show that in the United States, a firm handshake can make a good first impression with others, holding true for men and women, and so it is often explicitly taught.[13,14] Jennifer Cohen, a business consultant, describes the perfect handshake as having the following properties: The shaker should have good posture, make eye contact, hold the right hand out, give a good firm shake, hold for two seconds, smile, and greet the other person by name. She argues that this process conveys that the shaker is trustworthy, warm-spirited, confident, driven, and prepared.[15]

Handshakes in Medical Settings: The Physician

Prior to the pandemic, it was common for physicians to shake their patient's hand when entering the exam room. After shaking hands, the physician would then wash their hands or apply hand sanitizer and then sometimes put on exam gloves. A 2007 study asked patients how they would like to be greeted by their physicians, and most patients wanted their doctors to shake their hands, greet them by name, and introduce themselves, using their first and last names. Among respondents, 78% specifically stated that they wanted their doctor to shake their hand, underscoring the role of this ritual in establishing connection and trust. While shaking hands, respondents wanted their physicians to smile, be personable and attentive, and make eye contact, behaviors that communicated that the patient was a priority.[16]

The need for this ritualized exchange conflicts directly with the need to create and maintain a sterile field, but the motivations for and functionality of breaking sterility are understandable. In their unique fiduciary role, physicians are given distinctive access to our bodies when we are in particularly vulnerable states. We give them permission to touch us in places reserved for only the most intimate people in our lives when they must conduct certain procedures. Given the access that we might be asked to give them during an exam, it makes sense for physicians to start with a very common form of touch, such as a handshake or touch on the forearm. It provides a moment when the physician and the patient can start getting comfortable with the touch.[17]

We swallow the pills and extend our arms for injections. Patients are often in states of heightened anxiety, fear, and stress. Participating in the familiar act of handshaking, when done correctly, establishes a relationship of trust between physician and patient. The patient thinks, "I am a priority. I am in good, confident, trustworthy, and competent hands." First impressions are powerful and often have lasting impacts on relationships, and first impressions are made as we interpret verbal and nonverbal messages.

Even after the first interaction between doctor and patient, nonverbal communication continues to influence the interpretation of verbal messages, and patients distinguish between procedural touch requirements and comforting and communicative touches.[18,19] From the patient's perspective, comforting touches are those on the hand or forearm. Reassuring and supporting touches include help getting up from lying flat on an exam table.

Opportunities for nondiagnostic touch can also function to help temper physicians' tendency to view patients with a scientific gaze, as medical problems to be solved, and help them see their patients as complex beings navigating the world through their minds and bodies and as collections of lived experiences that will inform their experience of illness.[20] This tempering inevitably serves the physician and the patient.

Touch beyond the Handshake: Diagnosis

The handshake can establish an interaction, but beyond the handshake, touch is used in medical settings by doctors, nurses, and other allied professionals as a diagnostic and healing tool.

Consider the rich history of palpation as a core component of medical work. Physicians were taught to use touch to detect and diagnose numerous maladies before the advent of various blood tests and scanning procedures, from the X-ray to the ultrasound, CAT scan, and PET scan.[21] Palpation is a method of feeling the body with the fingers or hands to examine the size, consistency, texture, location, and tenderness of an organ or body part.[22] Physicians in the Middle Ages observed, palpated, felt the pulse, and visually examined urine as their limited but effective primary diagnostic tools.[23]

A physician's confident touches when palpating increases a patient's sense of the practitioner's competency. Too tentative a touch may increase anxiety, as a light touch might reveal the physician's insecurity. Too firm might cause significant pain and discomfort. Too firm might also be interpreted as aggressive, annoyed, or punitive.

Nurses' Touch

While the physician's touch is vital for communicating caring and competency during introduction, assessment, and treatment, by the nature of their work, nurses often have more frequent opportunities to touch their patients than do physicians, especially when we consider hospital-based nurses. While nurses' touches also convey caring and competency, the frequency and variety of situations where nurses touch patients create the context for a more complex function of touch in the nurse-patient interaction. In addition to caring and competent touches, nurses' touches help orient patients; allay fears and anxiety in situations when physicians are not present, but anxiety might be quite high (for example, before a procedure or in the middle of the night for the inpatient); and provide comfort.[24,25]

More on the Competent Touch

During the diagnostic and treatment stages for cancer patients, a competent touch from any variety of medical professionals provides numerous opportunities for relieving some of the patient's touch hunger, easing some of the inherent stress and anxiety associated with demanding treatments, and keeping the patient who is confronting their own mortality, who may be burdened by the physical pain and incapacities associated with their cancer, connected to the world.[26]

Let us consider a typical oncology appointment followed by an outpatient chemotherapy treatment. After checking in at the front desk, patients typically see the phlebotomist to get blood drawn (venipuncture). Many readers will have had the experience of having blood drawn even in the absence of any serious illness episodes. And those of us who have had multiple occasions for getting blood drawn will likely recall good and bad experiences.

A good experience begins with cordial introductions. After the patient is seated, the technician applies the tourniquet to increase pressure and make a vein more accessible. The touch of the preferred arm should be firm but not too firm, and the tourniquet feels necessarily tight, but ideally not painful. The phlebotomist's movements are fluid—no hesitation, no second-guessing. Once they identify a good vein, they adeptly insert the needle, and the process of collecting the samples, even if they need to change out a couple of tubes, is completed gracefully. The entire procedure flows like a well-orchestrated dance. The skill of their actions, the precision of their movements, exudes competence and self-confidence. The procedure seems to be over before it has even begun, and there is little evidence that blood was drawn later when the bandage is removed, other than the smallest mark where the needle was inserted.

A bad experience can begin with a stressed or otherwise unpleasant introduction. The tourniquet is much too tight. The technician's hesitation to set up the needles and tubes results in the tourniquet becoming increasingly, almost unbearably painful. There is no good vein, and somehow the patient may be made to feel as though this issue is a personal failing. Since a good vein is not identified, the needle misses it mark, sometimes more than once. What should be a graceful dance becomes a series of disjointed missteps. The patient's anxiety starts to swell as they lose confidence in the phlebotomist's skill. Later, bruising may be significant where the procedure was attempted. A bad venipuncture may set the stage for an unpleasant visit.

The next step is typically the collection of the vitals by members of the nursing staff. Again, this step ideally proceeds like a well-rehearsed dance. Weight and height are taken, basic questions reviewed, temperature and blood oxygen saturation recorded, and blood pressure measured with minimal discomfort. And, like the previous step, the entire process begins with a few shared kind words of introduction.

Touch during the measurement of vitals is far less direct than during the venipuncture. The most direct touch comes with the placement of the blood pressure cuff. Temperature is measured by a thermometer, oxygen by a pulse oximeter, weight and height by a scale. Technological tools substitute for the direct touch of the human hand, and the nurse's competency at this stage is assessed by the agility of the measurement processes and whether the way they ask basic questions about the patient's state of health communicates genuine interest in the answers.

These two steps are typically followed by the visit with the oncologist. The patient is escorted to an empty exam room, where they likely wait for some time for their oncologist. Once the oncologist enters the room, hopefully the desired handshake and introduction or greeting is offered, followed by the handwashing/sanitizing process. Based on what other tests have been done between visits, during this appointment, recent scans might be reviewed, or the oncologist reviews the latest blood tests and what they show. At this stage, the physician's primary role is to review test results and interpret data.

During my visits, after we reviewed scan and test results, my oncologist would have me get onto an exam table so that he could palpate my lymph nodes—neck, torso, and groin—and check the mobility of my right arm. He would always begin with me sitting up, and he would check the nodes in my neck. This moment was always oddly "close," as he would stand directly facing me, cupping my face in his hands, as he examined my nodes. This stance is one that outside medical settings we might associate with two intimates about to kiss, or the gesture of deep love or comfort communicated by a parent to their child. Cupping collapses the two individuals' focus on the person directly in front of them. During this moment, he would often ask me general questions about my life, I suspect to relieve some of the awkwardness of this very close stance. But this diagnostic touch was overlaid by an unintentional though welcomed touch of comfort, and I certainly knew that his focus was directly on me at that moment!

Once a patient lies back on the exam table, the prone position may leave them feeling vulnerable. It is also more likely that the physician is accessing parts of the body rarely touched by people outside a personal or familial tight circle. One of my personal quirks is that I have never liked having anyone touch my stomach, not even the most intimate people in my life, so whenever a physician has had a need to press on my belly, I am highly uncomfortable (but compliant). Once I was on my back and my oncologist was palpating my torso and groin, his questions would become more clinical—was there any discomfort or tenderness anywhere?

Once the palpation was complete, my oncologist would always help me sit up again. I did not need his help getting up (my core strength is still okay, despite my age), but I always appreciated this supportive touch. It helped relieve some of the anxiety I had before the physical exam had started, and it gave me a chance to be comforted before we would wrap up the exam and I would head off to my outpatient chemotherapy appointment.

Outpatient Chemotherapy and My Need for Touch

I talked about my outpatient chemotherapy experiences in Chapter 3, and I reference them again in later chapters, but here I want to address a particular experience from my third outpatient session that highlights the discussion of balancing the deep need for touch with the breaking of a sterile field.

I was just a few days past my inpatient methotrexate infusion, and I felt like a punching bag. I was once again in a treatment room without a window, which immediately dampened the mood before the infusion even began. I knew that the whole session would proceed more quickly since the team was less concerned about my having an allergic reaction to my cocktail, and there was comfort in this knowledge. My sister was once again with me, ready to provide whatever support I needed that day. But as hard as I wanted to be that "good patient," I was overwhelmed by knowing firsthand now everything that

I was about to experience—and that I absolutely did not want to experience. I did not want my port accessed, and I did not want the chemicals poured into my veins. I did not want to smell alcohol wipes or be hooked up to an IV stand. I felt like a petulant child who desperately needed a nap, and I started to cry. My sister, being there at the ready, held me tight until I could "just breathe."

What I did not know at that moment was that my main infusion nurse for the day was seeing this interaction and my tears. Instead of communicating impatience or frustration at the sight of a possibly unruly patient, she came into the room and asked, "Is this a hug day?" I told her about my extreme fatigue and anxiety, sharing the detail that I had just gotten out of the hospital two days earlier from my inpatient infusion.

At that moment, without a hint of hesitation or annoyance, she sterilized her hands, came over to me in my infusion chair, and gave me a huge hug. While hugging me, she told me that she was there for me and would be all day. My tears started flowing again, as this act of kindness and compassion was so incredibly lovely and much needed. But these tears were also cathartic, as I felt acknowledged without judgment and comforted. This oncology nurse, who was managing the care for a number of patients that day, was under no obligation to make this extra effort to comfort me, but this breaking of the barrier enabled me to reset and get ready for treatment. After our hug, she announced that she would sterilize herself again so we could begin. I was so incredibly grateful that she had broken the "barrier," and I also loved that she had sterilized her hands before she did!

Nursing has become a highly specialized profession, especially when you think of specific fields, such as oncology nursing. So during my interactions with nurses throughout my cancer experience, I simultaneously valued their displays of highly competent technical skills (accessing my port, administering the chemotherapy, managing my physical care) and their efforts to administer to my emotional and spiritual well-being.

Inpatient Infusions

Given the small but not zero risk that my lymphoma cells could cross the blood-brain barrier, in addition to my R-CHOP outpatient chemotherapy treatments, I had four inpatient methotrexate infusions since methotrexate is one of the few chemotherapy agents that crosses this barrier to prevent the development of a brain tumor. The treatment experience as an inpatient is qualitatively different than the outpatient experience, despite many commonalities. In this chapter, I explore some of the ways that the inpatient setting influences the treatment experience.

Methotrexate

In 1948, Sidney Farber discovered that aminopterin, a precursor to modern methotrexate, effectively led to remission in acute leukemias.[1] Methotrexate is in a class of medications called antimetabolites. Antimetabolites kill cells by mimicking the molecules that a cell needs to grow. Since antimetabolites are structurally very similar to metabolites (the basic components of our metabolism), dividing cells mistakenly use antimetabolites instead of the cells' own basic genetic material, RNA and DNA, to try to form new cells. Without the correct materials, these cells fail to reproduce and eventually die. Because antimetabolites target cells only as they are dividing, these medications are most effective against cells that are growing quickly, such as cancer cells.

To be effective at wiping out some aggressive cancer cells, such as lymphoma, methotrexate sometimes must be administered in high doses in an inpatient setting.[2] The factors that necessitate an inpatient infusion are multifold. Since cancer cells are not the only cells dividing at any time any chemotherapy agent is administered, care is taken to monitor and take measures to reduce the damage of the high dose on patients' healthy cells.[3] This goal is achieved in part by administering leucovorin, a drug that counters the impact of methotrexate.

After methotrexate interrupts the cancer cells' reproduction, it is removed by the kidneys and leaves the body in the urine. Full clearance of methotrexate can take several days, and during this time, patients are monitored for excessive damage to healthy cells and organs. Many factors affect how well one person's body clears methotrexate, and one quick clearance may not be followed by a quick clearance during the next infusion. But patients are not allowed to leave the hospital until the methotrexate has successfully cleared since delayed clearance can lead to lasting injury to the kidneys, mouth, digestive track, and immune system. They remain in the hospital and must have blood drawn to monitor the clearance. Since the toxin is removed via the kidneys and urine, inpatients are given IV fluids and are encouraged to drink as much water as they can tolerate. I had to keep track of my urine output during these inpatient infusions, to demonstrate that I was, in fact, continuing to drink water and to test whether my kidneys were functioning well. When high-dose methotrexate is given, the kidneys work harder than normal to clear it, so it is especially important to keep the kidneys functioning.

The Hospital as a Total Institution

The reasons why high-dose methotrexate is best administered in an inpatient setting are understandable, given the simultaneous need for a high dose and the danger of uncontrolled toxicity. But the inpatient experience, while sharing some aspects of the outpatient experience, is a more immersive and controlling environment, and it illustrates aspects of Erving Goffman's description of a "total institution."

In his 1968 book, *Asylums*, Goffman defines total institutions to identify and analyze how they are different from other institutional settings.[4] Examples of total institutions include prisons, mental institutions, and monasteries. What separates total institutions from other modern institutions are some shared characteristics. While most people in modern society work and sleep in two separate settings, differentiating between their work/professional lives and their personal/family lives, institutionalized individuals combine these two spheres within the total institutional setting. "Work" and "personal" activities are experienced under the rule of a single authority, and the institutionalized members of the total institution are typically required to engage in the same activities for a shared aim. Even if we consider the few previous examples of total institutions, we see that the shared aim between different kinds of total institutions can vary significantly, even if they share these characteristics. For example, the aims or functions of the prison can be multifold. We might propose that some of the functions include protecting the wider society from a dangerous criminal, (ideally) rehabilitating the individual, repairing the damage caused by the criminal act by defining some punishment, and deterring future criminal acts. The functions of the mental institution may include protecting the committed individual against self-harm or harm to others and (ideally) helping the individual "get better" and resume their normal activities. We might propose that one of the functions of the monastery is providing clerics with a way to remove themselves from the distractions of the world to focus on their religious devotion. The process for joining the total institution may be involuntary (prisons), voluntary (monastery), or a combination of both (mental institution).

I discussed another aspect of the process of joining a total institution in Chapter 2 when talking about patients' adoption of the sick role—the stripping of the former identity and the donning of the "uniform" associated with the new role. The prisoner wears the prison uniform, the mental patient wears the patient robes and clothes assigned to them, and the monk or cleric wears the robes designating their order. Aspects of personal identity are stripped to create a new identity as an "inmate" of the new institution. The stripping of the personal identity is also accompanied by restrictions on self-determination. In total institutions, inmates often follow strict schedules that are enforced by a central authority.

The patient admitted to the hospital is exposed to some of the same restrictions and experiences of the inmates in the total institutions discussed earlier, but hopefully at a far less lengthy and extreme degree. As previously noted, they may be stripped of their normal clothing and asked to wear the patient gown. During their stay, they are conducting almost all their daily activities within the confines of the hospital and under the control of their medical team. They are often on floors and in wards with people with similar medical conditions, all who might be experiencing similar treatment plans with the shared aim of getting better.

Numerous restrictions are placed on a patient's self-determination. The patient typically cannot request or control the room to which they are assigned. They cannot control who is assigned to them for their nursing care. They are not able to control the timing of their meals or the timing of the taking of their vitals or of their treatments. While each of these disruptions might seem minor, together they can create significant stress for the patient and lead to what Goffman describes as the mortification of the self, or the loss of self-esteem and self-identity.[4,5] We often do not consider how important certain daily routines might be in our expression of self until they are taken away—the morning cup of coffee at the table while reading the newspaper, the walk around the neighborhood, the lunch at noon sharp, or the flexibility to have lunch whenever we are hungry. We might also not realize how participating in these routines provides opportunities for self-expression and for exercising our independence and autonomy. For example, few patients tell their nurses that they refuse to have their vitals taken at 5:00 A.M. since it is inconvenient or interrupts their sleep. Some do, but they risk being viewed as bad or uncooperative patients.

My Total Institution Experiences

Windowless Rooms and One Hallway

During my first inpatient infusion, I was assigned to a room on the hospital's oncology "overflow" floor, and I had a roommate. Since 2019, the University of Pennsylvania has built a new hospital that has only single rooms. In 2019, while there were special oncology floors with windows and singles in newer sections of the "old" hospital, they were often booked to capacity, given the volume of patients who were admitted for cancer treatments at the Hospital of the University of Pennsylvania (HUP), and so my first draw was on this overflow floor.

The room was very cramped. It had two hospital beds with the classic curtain between, and then each "side" had one additional chair for one visitor. You had to squeeze between the visitor's chair and the patient bed on side A to access side B. Since my roommate and I were admitted for an inpatient infusion, we also had to navigate around the room with our IV poles.

The windows on the floor were all frosted, and this wing of the hospital was constructed very close to another tall building, so there was basically no natural light. I was assigned to side A, and only side B had even one frosted window. While in my hospital bed during this first infusion, there was no way for me to track the passing of time except by checking my cell phone or my Fitbit. The total lack of natural light was terribly disorienting.

As noted earlier, we were highly encouraged to walk as much as possible during our inpatient stays. Walking helped the body clear out the methotrexate and prevent other side effects related to being even temporarily inactive, such as boosting mood, increasing appetite and aiding in digestion, and helping patients sleep. Aiding appetite and digestion was especially important, given that methotrexate causes nausea.

In my attempt to fulfill the role of "good patient," I walked the hallway multiple times every day. The challenge during this first inpatient assignment was the fact that the hallway was short and incredibly limited: no windows and only about ten rooms long. At each end of the hallway were two thick double doors that separated the floor at one end from a main hospital hallway and at the other end from another section of the hospital. You could leave the hallway if you got permission, but this excursion was discouraged by the nursing staff, especially for patients receiving their methotrexate infusions for the first time (since they were uncertain how patients might respond). So, walk this limited hall I did, dragging my IV pole. By the end of the first day, I felt overly familiar with the different pieces of "art" adorning the hallway's walls.

No Uniform and Some Comfort Items!

Unlike Goffman's classic total institutions, in 2019 at HUP, cancer patients admitted for inpatient infusions were allowed to wear whatever clothes they wanted, as long as the clothes permitted easy access to ports or peripherally inserted central catheter (PICC) lines.[6] The traditional patient gown was not a forced uniform. Patients were also encouraged to bring other kinds of comforting or helpful items, such as special blankets, pillows, books, Internet devices, water bottles, and so forth. These measures helped mitigate the mortification of the self during admission, as they let patients retain and express their personal identities and self-determination.

Most inpatients on the floor tended to wear very comfortable clothing— very loose tops and pants. Depending on the stage of their treatment, some patients wore wigs or scarves, while others did not bother with any head coverings. Few patients wore traditional pajamas, I suspect because of the 24/7 nature of the floor experience. While lights were dimmed from about 10:00 P.M. until about 6:00 A.M., all patients were routinely interrupted during the night for taking vitals, changing IV bags, and administering chemotherapy, so in practice no differentiation between daytime and nighttime activities was marked by the changing of a "uniform." And since we were all hooked up to IV poles, changing clothes, especially tops, was not easy! When changing IV lines, I always appreciated when the nurses gave me a chance to put on different clothes, freshen up with a washcloth, or go to the bathroom free from the IV pole.

An example of the 24/7 nature of the cancer ward is well illustrated by aspects of the methotrexate infusion. Given the toxic capability of methotrexate, the infusion is tightly controlled. A particular detail of the process includes monitoring the pH level of patients' urine. As noted earlier, the kidneys are primarily responsible for removing the methotrexate once it has had the time to interrupt the cancer cells' division. Methotrexate is a dicarboxylic acid that is soluble in human blood, which normally has a pH level of 7.35 to 7.45 (slightly alkaline or basic).[7,8] But to keep the drug from forming crystals (taking a "solid" form) during its removal by the kidneys, patients' urine, which has a wide normal pH range from 4.5 to 8, must be kept "basic," with a pH level of 7.5 or greater.[9] Patients' urine must test as basic before the infusion can begin. This result is facilitated by administering sodium bicarbonate—good ol' baking soda—until the urine's pH registers at ≥7.5. My oncologist had me take sodium bicarbonate orally (pills) before my inpatient admissions, and then I would finish the process hooked up to a sodium bicarbonate IV.

It was hard to predict when the urine would finally hit the right number so that the infusion could begin. As a patient, you want it to begin as soon as possible because the sooner it starts, the sooner you can begin the recovery/removal process and get out of the hospital. But since the normal range is so wide and so many different factors can affect the urine's pH level, what might be achieved in a few hours during one admission might take almost twelve hours to achieve on another visit. It also depended on the time that you were admitted; an early admission might mean starting the infusion right after lunch, but a late afternoon or evening admission might mean not reaching the target number until 1:00 A.M.

On more than one occasion, I hit my target urine pH after normal working hours. The first time this happened, I learned that the on-site hospital pharmacy was staffed 24/7 precisely so that patients' treatments could be prepared in the middle of the night, if necessary. I desperately wanted to tell the pharmacy team how much I appreciated their being on call so that I would not have to wait until the next morning to start the treatment.

The contents of the overnight bag that I brought to the hospital for each inpatient admission changed over time as I learned what additional comforting items I needed for the inpatient stays, but they always included an unbelievably soft dark blue plush blanket (given to me by my eldest before my first admission); my laptop computer; my cell phone; a few different books and magazines, as I was never sure what mood I might be in (would I be in the mood for comedy, fiction, or perhaps science fiction and/or horror?); and a twenty-ounce, double-walled, stainless-steel insulated travel tumbler. The tumbler made all the difference for me, as I am a huge fan of iced drinks, and the tumbler made it possible to always have access, day or night, to a very cold drink. Later on, I also learned the significant benefit of bringing a tube or tub of Aquaphor since my outpatient and inpatient chemotherapy protocols resulted in cracked or peeling skin, especially on my hands.[10]

Food

Few people are likely to be excited by the prospect of ordering hospital meals. As this inpatient stay was not my first in my life, I was well aware that hospital fare was about as appetizing as that of most institutional food services, such as college dining centers. I had very low expectations, but I also had a very limited appetite, as I already suffered persistent nausea from the R-CHOP treatments. It still was a bit fun (and a distraction) to read the daily hospital menu and try to imagine what I might possibly enjoy for any one of the daily meals. At the time, HUP's menu included some daily specials, which made the process even more entertaining.

While the food was never worthy of a star rating, I did greatly appreciate the people who took the food orders. They were kind and patient, I suspect in part because they understood that cancer patients were likely managing significant intestinal distress and nausea. I always welcomed their visit, as they were among the few hospital employees who were not there to poke me or measure some bodily function.

I learned during that first visit that each oncology floor was equipped with a special communal kitchen where patients had access to refrigerator space and a variety of frozen meals, snacks, and drinks. My reaction was a deep sense of gratitude. In recognition of the sometimes-severe side effects from treatment, this resource gave patients the opportunity to eat whenever they could manage if nausea and vomiting prevented them from eating at regular mealtimes. This structural flexibility reduced the regimentation that would have resulted from having meals provided only within institutionally defined and enforced time frames, thereby lessening the "total institution" feel of the inpatient stay.

Access to space in the refrigerator also made it possible to bring food from home as an alternative to or supplement for the hospital food. As the side effects seemed to accumulate over the months of treatment, this benefit was huge. Another side effect from a wide range of chemotherapy agents coupled with reduced physical activity during an inpatient stay is constipation. Numerous times during inpatient stays, I had to take stool softeners, as patients had to successfully evacuate before they could be discharged. The great benefit of being able to bring food from home meant that I could pack very high-fiber foods that I knew I would enjoy and would help prevent constipation. They often included very high-fiber soups (for example, bean-based soups) that I found I could often tolerate even when nauseated. Akin to wearing my own clothes, bringing my own food helped mitigate self-mortification and enhance self-determination.

Visitors

Visitors provide a vital connection to the "outside" world for the inpatient. Family members, friends, and even occasionally coworkers are among those who visit the inpatient, and they help keep the patient linked to at least some of their non-sick roles. Visitors provide needed familiar company, communicate news about people outside the hospital, and help pass time for inpatients stripped of their normal roles and activities.

Unlike those who enter a monastery, the inpatient enters the hospital with the intention of limiting their time at the institution as much as possible. The goal of admission is to stabilize, treat, and/or restore the patient to their preadmission state of health. It is in the interest of the patient and of the hospital to limit the duration since unnecessary days may increase the chance of hospital-acquired patient complications, such as secondary infections, and add to the eventual costs for patients and healthcare systems.[11]

In the United States, the average length of a hospital stay for all medical conditions combined is around five days. For cancer patients, the average is 6.5 days, in part because of the negative side effects of treatment, including but not limited to rendering the patient acutely immunocompromised. The average cost per day for hospitalization for all conditions combined is $2,800, while for cancer patients, the cost is $3,400.[12]

We might think that a week is not a very long time to be separated from your normal routines and, therefore, that visits might be less important for keeping the patient connected to their normal social roles. But we need to consider the anxiety and fear the cancer patient might be experiencing in addition to the punishing aspects of treatment. Connection and distraction are very important.

Disoriented

As previously noted, the inpatient experience can be disorienting for many reasons—separation from normal routines, potential lack of natural light, and a 24/7 treatment schedule are just a few examples. This feeling is why mealtimes can gain extra meaning for patients—they help anchor the daily clock. But perhaps the most disorienting feature is the regular change of the staff taking care of patients. At least twice a day, the oncology nurse overseeing their care changes, and this switch basically marks the difference between day and night. Not only does the primary oncology nurse change; so does the ancillary nursing staff who assist the oncology nurses. These are the staff members who regularly take vitals and help with communication and some basic care, but not with accessing ports or PICCs for infusions.

Like many hospital systems, HUP provided whiteboards in the room to make it easier for patients to keep track of this regular changing of the guard. Ideally, as each new staff member started their shift, they wrote their name on the whiteboard, large enough so that the patient could easily read it from their bed (especially important for older patients, who might have diminished eyesight). The whiteboards at HUP had spaces for about eight different staff members with whom the patient might interact, but typically, only the head nurse's name made it onto the board. HUP also posted pictures of a patient's nurse on their door, which helped connect names and faces.

Sometimes I would see the same nurse for the same shift for two days in a row, but this occurrence was less frequent than I would have hoped. Seeing a familiar face was very comforting and freed me from having to "get to know" someone new so often, even during one stay. And I wanted to get to know each of my nurses, so with every change, I made an effort to touch base with them in very basic ways. This desire was driven by my personality and by my status as a sociologist, as mentioned before. But it was often driven, especially in the inpatient setting, by my recognition of my intense reliance on these professionals to successfully manage this infusion. Rightly or wrongly, the sheer fact that this treatment could not be done as an outpatient procedure made me feel more vulnerable than I felt during any of my R-CHOP outpatient treatments. I wanted to know something about the person in whose hands I would be for the next twelve hours of my life.

Although I already have sung the praises of some of my outpatient nurses, I want to give a special shout-out here to the entire nursing staff who took care of me as an inpatient and an outpatient at HUP. Of all the nurses and nursing assistants with whom I interacted over the months of treatment, I did not have confidence in only one nurse. During inpatient and outpatient infusions, cancer patients are cared for by the oncology nursing staff. Physicians do make rounds at the hospital, but the nurses are administering the treatments and monitoring the entire process, 24/7. They are accessing the ports and PICCs, starting the lines, managing all the tests, and coordinating every treatment and posttreatment protocol. As discussed in Chapter 9, the display of caring and competency by medical professionals is highly valued by patients. The display of caring and competency by the oncology nurses is essential when you watch them access your ports and PICCs and hook you up to the dangerous chemicals that hopefully will save your life. My nursing staff regularly presented as confident and, therefore, competent. They were kind whether working on me at 3:00 P.M. or at 3:00 A.M. And whenever they had a question or concern, they reached out for support from their colleagues.

I had one nurse (who took care of me twice while I was an inpatient) who was not a "fan" of my particular port, the PowerPort. She had had trouble accessing it on a previous patient, and it had not been a pleasant experience for either of them. Since this experience had happened recently, she was not confident to try to access my port, as she did not want to start out my inpatient experience with a potentially unpleasant incident. She was honest about admitting her own hesitation and recruited one of her colleagues to access my port.[13] Instead of decreasing my confidence in her, her honesty and desire to protect me increased my belief that I was indeed in very good hands.

Nighttime

While I have suggested that there is little difference between the day and night shifts other than the dimming of the lights, some experiential differences occur for patients and staff, even though many activities of the floor continue unchanged. In Eviatar Zerubavel's book *Patterns of Time in Hospital Life*, he analyzes the 24/7 nature of hospital life and the impact of this 24/7 experience, primarily on hospital staff.[14] Specifically, he notes a greater sense of solidarity among the night staff, noting that the "temporal roles" of working the overnight shift deepen relationships between staff members beyond the bonds they already share due to common professional roles. Violating the "normal clock" creates space for connection and communication between staff that would be less likely to occur during a normal daytime shift.

I would extend this argument to interactions between patients and staff members, especially for patients whose treatment includes multiple inpatient stays. Being an inpatient more than once increases the chance that patients will see some staff members again and that they will develop a familiarity with the floor/ward. Throughout human history, kings, poets, laborers, and children have noted that nighttime sets the stage for fretting and for asking existential questions about the human experience. Patients and staff are likely to find themselves facing some existential questions together in the middle of the night.

How common is nighttime fretting? Research by the American Academy of Sleep Medicine found that nearly 90% of Americans had lost sleep at night in 2022 due to worries about the economy and health.[15] While the study found that 87% of people lost sleep while worrying about money, worries about health kept 86% of people up at night, with 65% reporting specific concerns about the COVID-19 pandemic. But why at night? When we turn out the lights and all is dark and quiet, nothing distracts us from our internal thoughts. We are released from the daytime obligations whose distractions help keep our anxieties at bay.

Experts have found that regular bedtime routines can help people sleep better. A quick Google search shows many sites with lists of suggested pre-bedtime routines. A Healthline site offers twenty-three (!) suggestions, while a site sponsored by the Mayo Clinic narrows them down to six core practices: (1) Stick to a sleep schedule, (2) pay attention to what you eat and drink, (3) create a restful environment, (4) limit daytime naps, (5) include physical activity in your daily routine, and (6) manage worries.[16,17] But if we consider for a moment the experience of the hospitalized cancer patient, even Mayo's most basic suggestions seem unachievable. Numerous studies have documented the sleep challenges faced by hospitalized patients: diminished total sleep time, abnormal sleep architecture (that is, disruption in normal patterns of

REM [rapid eye movement] and non-REM sleep), and multiple awakenings by staff or by environmental noise and lights.[18,19] Hospitalized patients also report challenges associated directly with illness, such as pain.[20] In addition to these challenges, cancer patients have significant trouble trying to adhere to routines associated with eating and drinking (due to nausea), getting adequate physical activity, and, perhaps most tricky, managing their worries. Inpatient sleep disruptions, however, can negatively affect patients' physical, emotional, and cognitive statuses, thereby impairing patients' overall sense of well-being. The more items that patients can bring to the hospital to help create a comforting and familiar environment (such as my blue plush blanket or a favorite pillow), the better.

During my inpatient stays, I had my share of fretful nights, either because of treatment, nausea, or just rampant anxiety. So, when I was awake or had to be woken up for care, I appreciated the opportunity to share some middle-of-the-night conversations with staff members.

The nurses were always remarkably gentle if they had to wake me up in the middle of the night. I appreciated this care immensely, as ever since I was a young child, I have always been startled if woken up. On other occasions, the staff found me awake when making their general rounds and would take a moment to see whether I needed anything. During these midnight-hour interactions, the staff seemed less rushed than during the day, in part because at least some of their patients were asleep, so they did have an extra minute or two to spare. Especially when they found me alone, frightened, anxious, and unable to sleep, we shared stories that provided great comfort, a connection to the world outside the hospital, and the needed distraction so that I eventually could get some sleep.

One of the most common topics of these late-night conversations was the reason(s) they had pursued careers in healthcare. As a medical sociologist, I was professionally interested in these stories, but as the person currently in their care, I was also personally intrigued. How did this person come to be by my hospital bedside in the middle of the night? The stories were as rich and diverse as the individuals in my room. One young woman decided to pursue oncology nursing after she had lost her mother to cancer in high school. She was inspired by the nurses who took such loving care of her mother and wanted to give back. Several of them were following in family members' footsteps. All spoke about how they could not imagine doing anything other than what they were doing, how they had always felt a calling to nursing, how the field fascinated and fulfilled them.

A few of them also told me about how being a nurse was helping or had helped them raise their families, given the flexibility of scheduling. If I learned that they had children, we had a whole new topic for conversation! Tell me about your children, and I will tell you about mine. How old are they? What do they do? And they would tell me lovely stories and make me laugh.

During these inpatient stays, I was reading *The Fifth Season* and *The Obelisk Gate* by N. K. Jemisin.[21,22] One nurse was also reading these books, and we spent some time talking about the series, sharing notes, and recommending other science fiction writers.

What none of them ever did was try to tell me that everything was going to be okay, that I was fine, and that my worries were unwarranted. If I needed to share my fears in the middle of the night—or one time, in the afternoon—they listened. I suspected that as frontline workers, they knew that not every patient at whose bedside they stood would make it. They may have been able to make some pretty good predictions based on the treatment responses that they saw every day, but they might have been surprised enough over the course of their careers at who did and who did not achieve remission that they avoided potentially overly optimistic generalizations. And I appreciated that. I do not want to suggest that they just left my expression of fear hanging out there. They acknowledged the fear and then asked me what they could do, right at that moment, to help. Sometimes that meant squeezing my hand. Other times, it meant getting me some Zofran and filling my tumbler with ice and fresh water. At times, it was allowing me to cry for a few moments before they accessed my port. And sometimes, it was simply the offer to listen for a few moments, even if I did not want to talk. The midnight hours can be filled with angst, but they can also be filled with great kindness.

Roommates and Some Problematic Behavior

As noted earlier, when I was assigned to the overflow floor at HUP for my first and second inpatient infusions, I had a roommate. For my second admission, I was assigned to the exact same bed in the exact same room—what were the odds of that happening? For my last two inpatient infusions, I had a "single" on the regular oncology floor.

Hospitals all over the nation are transitioning to single-patient rooms in an effort to improve clinical outcomes, especially infection, and to comply with Health Insurance Portability and Accountability Act regulations.[23,24] In the near future, having a hospital roommate is likely to become a rare event.

During my first two inpatient infusions, having a roommate was simultaneously a comfort and a challenge.

My first roommate was a lovely woman, about my age, being treated for leukemia. She had a lovely hearty laugh, even though she was suffering from pretty extreme nausea. It was comforting to share a room for the first inpatient admission so that I could get some "tips" from someone who had been through the process already. She gave me the inside scoop on how to order from the hospital menu, and she shared her views on PICC lines versus ports (she had decided to just stick with a PICC). It was nice to be able to directly access a patient's perspective during the first day and night. And she graciously allowed me to ask as many questions as I needed.

The challenge of this first roommate was her particular coping method: To fully distract herself from her cancer, the treatment, and her fears, she immersed herself in crime dramas. All day and all night, she watched crime dramas on her TV without headphones. All day and all night, the room was filled with the background noise of blood-curdling screams, gunshots, and car chases. The first night, at around midnight, when the TV was still on, I asked my nurse for some earplugs and made a note that I should bring earplugs for the next admission. This roommate was discharged after two days, and as she was leaving, she left a true crime novel for me to read.

Within twelve hours, my first roommate was replaced with another woman, about fifteen years younger than I, who also had leukemia. She was a lawyer. She was tall and the best overall description would be elegant. She was one of the few patients who wore a wig in the hospital, and the wig gave her an appearance of health that was deceiving. But when she was walking around, heading to our shared bathroom, taking a walk down the hall, or even navigating our cramped room with her IV pole, she still looked elegant.

My second roommate was less conversive than my first, and in part a result of her husband's constant presence. While I had daily visits from my husband, and periodic visits from my children and from my sister, her husband basically never left the hospital. She was just less available for the spontaneous conversation. He actually shared her hospital bed overnight, much to the dismay of the nurses taking care of her (there was a reclining chair that he could have used but did not). I found their bed-sharing dear and a little unnerving, even though they were behind a curtain! I had no say in observing even indirectly this act of intimacy.

My roommate for the second admission on the overflow floor was a woman my age whose leukemia had spread to her brain. She was receiving methotrexate to address the spread. This was her seventh admission. She was very gregarious with me, and her husband spent most of the day with her, as he was already retired. She was far more talkative than her husband, who seemed somewhat henpecked. She told me that at that point, she never ate the hospital food and regularly sent him out to pick up food from one of the many restaurants bordering the hospital (near the University of Pennsylvania campus). She also bragged about how much she walked every day at the hospital. But her bravado could not fully hide her fear. She confessed to me in the middle of the night that she was terrified since the cancer had spread to her brain.

While she was pleasant to me and to my visitors, she did not treat everyone at the hospital well. While she was perfectly amiable with the rounding physicians, she was less kind to the nurses and outright unkind to support staff, especially to the phlebotomists and the hospital food staff. I suspected that her callous behavior with these staff members stemmed from her fear. Bullying them gave her some sense of control in what clearly was a terrifying situation. She repeatedly called the nurses, even when they explained that she was not due for any medication, and argued that according to her notes, she was due. She complained that every phlebotomist was incompetent and had hurt her. But her treatment of the food staff was in some ways the most inexplicable. As stated, she did not eat the hospital food, but she ordered food for every meal and gave the staff collecting the orders a hard time by making numerous special requests for each meal. If the food was late according to her sense of when breakfast, lunch, or dinner should be served, she "sent it back," arguing that it was no longer appropriate. She complained that her tea was cold and that her ice cream had melted, even though she already had sent her husband out an hour before for fresh coffee and donuts. This performance was so demonstrative that she immediately secured her reputation as "difficult," and when a food staff member came into the room, they rolled their eyes at me. The nurses also shook their heads and sighed as they came into our room.

This roommate and my elegant roommate also challenged some of the floor rules, which caused problems for the nursing staff. My elegant roommate got us into trouble by using the public bathroom instead of the bathroom assigned to us in the room. Since cancer patients are expelling toxic chemotherapy agents via their urine, we were given explicit instructions to use only our own bathroom and to have any visitor use the public bathrooms to protect against their accidental exposure to toxic agents. But as I also mentioned, we were drinking water excessively as well as receiving IV fluids, so we visited the bathroom quite often! There were numerous times when I had to pee but had to wait for my roommate to finish. She decided that she did not want to wait for me to finish one time and went out to the public bathroom. Her visit contaminated the public space, and the nurses had to call environmental services to come clean the public bathroom. When she was reprimanded, she said that she would do it again if she had to pee and I was in the bathroom. They responded by getting her a portable commode. This exchange played out like a game of chicken. Later that evening, my roommate explained that she was just so incredibly tired of following all the rules and restrictions from months of treatment and weeks upon weeks in the hospital. She never used the portable commode, and she never used the public bathroom again while we shared the room.

As mentioned earlier, my other roommate boasted about how much walking she did, and she challenged the nurses by leaving the floor to walk around the hospital without getting permission to leave. They came looking for her, realized that she had left, and then requested via the public announcement system that she return. They explained to her that they needed to know where she was in case she experienced any adverse events due to the methotrexate treatment, but she chuckled that she knew her way around.

Two for One—Tooth Extraction and Methotrexate

Hair follicles, skin cells, and the cells that line the gastrointestinal tract, including those in the mouth, are some of the fastest-growing cells in the human body and, therefore, very sensitive to the effects of chemotherapy, resulting in mouth sores and tooth infections.[25] As nausea and vomiting are common side effects from treatment, the development of any oral maladies exacerbates the problems cancer patients face when trying to eat during treatment.

Right before my second inpatient admission, I developed an infection in my left back lower molar. This tooth had been causing me problems since the birth of my son in 1994. During that pregnancy, I loss some bone mass in my jaw right around that tooth. Some bone loss is a common experience during and right after pregnancy due to the competing nutrient demands of the host and the developing fetus.[26] Some bone loss may be permanent. Nearly 60%–75% of pregnant women also develop gingivitis, an early stage of periodontal disease that occurs when the gums become red and swollen from inflammation that results from changing hormones during pregnancy.[27] Since 1994, this particular molar had "wiggled" a bit, and my dentist cleaned the area extra carefully each time I had my dental cleanings—we were trying to hold onto it for as long as possible—but the final assault and subsequent loss of the tooth came two months into my treatment. There was no saving the tooth at that point—it would have to be extracted.

There are added complications treating dental problems while under treatment for cancer since chemotherapy can leave patients immunocompromised. Many dental procedures, even basic cleanings, can cause bleeding of the gums. Bleeding provides a path for bacteria from the mouth to easily access the bloodstream. While the person with a functioning immune system typically would be able to manage this bacterial load, the immunocompromised patient might not, so treating dental problems during cancer treatment becomes a balance between managing the problem and minimizing infection risk.[28]

Anyone who has experienced an infected tooth likely remembers that the associated pain is far worse than the actual risk the tooth poses to an individual's overall health. The pain is extreme. When I first felt the tooth and knew that something was significantly wrong, my dentist got me an emergency appointment with an oral surgeon. This surgeon knew that I was immunocompromised and that I would be going in shortly for my second inpatient infusion, so he got on the phone with the oral surgeons at HUP to see whether I could get a "two-procedures-for-one-admission" special. He argued that having the folks at Penn take the tooth while I was getting my methotrexate would be the best way to control my infection risk from the procedure. I just had to wait a few days to get relief.

I was in significant pain from the infected molar when I was admitted and learned from my nurses that I could not take Tylenol or Aleve for the pain since these medications could mask a fever, and my team needed to know whether I ran a fever during the infusion. So, instead of these common, over-the-counter meds, I was given a low dose of morphine. Morphine is an opioid that works directly on the opioid receptors in the brain, blocking pain messages.[29] Morphine is also a central nervous system depressant, a type of drug that slows down brain activity, so in addition to blocking pain, it also can render a patient sleepy and a bit dopey, but until the tooth was removed, it was the only way I was going to be able to control the extreme pain.[30] Luckily, my infection was very localized— there was no suggestion of a more systemic infection or the involvement of more than that one tooth. For example, my #18 molar hurt like the dickens, but I could tap #19 with no pain at all. I reported the average pain of #18 as an 8 on a scale of 1–10. I was visited for a few days prior to the procedure by several members of the oral surgery staff. Every day for the next few days, dental residents would come in and tap #18 and the surrounding teeth, and I would report every time that it hurt like hell (even with the morphine). We well established which tooth was the problem.

The morphine made it hard to keep up with my regular strolls up and down the hall since I was so sleepy, and that limitation significantly affected my infusion experience. Since movement helps the body expel the methotrexate, the ideal is to get it out of your body as quickly as possible after twenty-four hours. As a central nervous system depressant, morphine slows down messages from the brain to a variety of organ systems, resulting in slower movement of muscles, and it also slows down digestion and excretion (resulting in constipation). I was caught between a rock and a hard place. I started my methotrexate drip on a Friday, but I did not have the tooth removed until Monday, so for a little more than two days, I had to trade off pain control and sleeping against walking and proper functioning of the systems that would pass the drug. It was very unpleasant, and I experienced some of the worse nausea and constipation of my life.

The tooth extraction went relatively easily. Once I finally got into the chair and settled, it seemed to take less than a minute to pull the tooth from my jaw. It was a painful procedure, but the oral surgery resident who took the tooth and I were grateful that it was not complicated.

Despite the relative ease of the actual extraction, when I got back to my room, my body dissented. Between the methotrexate flowing through my body and the tooth extraction, my body decided that enough was enough and that it was going into shutdown mode. Even on the wheelchair ride back to my room, I started to shake like one does when they have a fever, but I did not have a fever. I did not want anyone to touch me for quite some time—not to comfort me, nor take my vitals, nothing. All my body wanted to do was sleep. My husband covered me with my dark blue plush blanket, I closed my eyes, and I shook under the covers, avoiding everyone.

By Tuesday morning, the chills had fully passed, but I was still feeling quite knocked down. That morning, the oncology nurse practitioner came to review my blood work. She reported that my methotrexate level was still too high for me to be released, my white blood counts were too low, and unfortunately, my liver numbers were a bit elevated, suggesting that my liver was being affected by the infusion. I started to cry, as all I wanted to do was go home, sleep in my own bed, look out the window at natural light. Dismayed by my crying, she spiritedly added, "Your kidneys look great!" This addition made me laugh, even though I knew that they were going to keep me and reassess my numbers on Wednesday.

Thankfully, this dental complication was the only one beyond mouth sores that I experienced for the rest of my treatment.

A Room with a View

For my last two admissions, I scored a single, private room on an upper floor of the hospital, with views overlooking the University of Pennsylvania campus. I was giddy when they showed me to my room at the start of my third admission. The addition of natural light made the experience much more bearable, as did the extra space to navigate about the room. Getting to and from the bathroom was much easier, and I no longer had to share the bathroom with a roommate. While it was beneficial not to have to listen to someone else's TV choices, it was also a bit unnerving not to have another person in the room with whom to share spontaneous conversations.

Unlike in my room on the overflow floor, I could spend most of my waking hours in a very comfortable chair or walking about the floor. Not having to spend the vast majority of my time in a bed was a huge improvement. This floor was organized as a large rectangle. When you first come onto the floor from the elevators, you are greeted at the front nursing desk. Then, the patient rooms are all on the perimeter of the floor, with each one having at least one window. A hallway cuts through the middle of the rectangle, and the rooms without windows include storage rooms, a conference room, and the communal kitchen. I was so invigorated by the layout because it meant that on this floor, I could walk laps rather than walking up and down one hallway! And when I got tired of walking in one direction, I could turn around and walk in the other direction! And if I wanted to make the lap a little shorter, I could cut through the central hallway.

Despite these wonderful, improved amenities, by the third admission, I was beginning to feel the accumulated wear and tear of the combined outpatient and inpatient infusions. Being constantly bound to an IV pole was becoming almost intolerable, and the methotrexate seemed to have more substantial negative side effects with each infusion. I would feel like I had just gotten ahead of the fatigue from the outpatient R-CHOP infusion, and then I would be scheduled to head back in for an inpatient infusion and get slammed with a new wave of fatigue. The nausea was also more severe, though bringing some high-fiber food from home made it easier to manage the nausea and the constipation.

Another new development at this stage of treatment was my sensitivity to the smells and sounds of the hospital. The smell of antiseptic wipes, the beeps of the machines started to trigger feelings of nausea even before anyone had started a procedure. This reaction was incredibly unpleasant, as there was no way to avoid these smells and sounds.

Trying to Stay Active

Posters reminding/encouraging admitted patients to remain active to make their treatment as effective and as least damaging as possible hang in every patient room and on the hallways. While this activity is the ideal, with each admission, I found it harder to move as much as I was encouraged to. While I was quite active before my diagnosis and tried my best to stay active while in treatment, this movement became increasingly challenging, primarily due to extreme fatigue.

What percentage of the adult U.S. population gets the recommended levels of physical activity, not considering a cancer diagnosis? When assessing general health-related recommendations, we must first recognize that they change over time and by age. Remember, physicians once recommended that people smoke![31] What might have been recommended fifty years ago will be modified based on people's working conditions (degrees to which people are doing manual labor versus desk/office labor) and their eating habits (for example, how many calories we consume on average every day).

According to the current CDC and the U.S. Department of Health and Human Services recommendations, adults in the United States need 150 minutes of moderate-intensity physical activity and two days of muscle-strengthening activity per week.[32] Despite this recommendation, only about 47% of U.S. adults get this much physical activity, and only about 24% meet the physical-activity and the muscle-strengthening goals.[33]

So, how much physical activity does the cancer patient need? In 2022, the American Society of Clinical Oncology officially recommended that patients also get 150 minutes, with a target of 30 minutes a day, five days a week—no different than the average American adult.[34] This recommendation came after a review of numerous studies that showed that physical activity during treatment was associated with higher survival rates and better responses to treatment. But a 2017 study found that about 75% of people reduce their exercise post-diagnosis, with only 16% maintaining their current levels and 4% increasing their levels.[35] We only need to recall any of the numerous side effects from treatment to understand why it might be hard for patients to be active. As already mentioned, the fatigue is brutal, but there is also the nausea and the time consumed by treatment, and we should not underestimate the impact of sadness and anxiety.

I found it much easier to keep moving when I was not in the hospital, as I was always motivated to get my dogs out for a walk. But even later in the treatment process, I would often find myself collapsing into a chair in my living room and not moving after getting back from one of my walks. When I was admitted, treatment fatigue was increased not only by the methotrexate but by sleep being interrupted in the middle of the night by the treatment protocol. A typical night in the hospital included being interrupted at 11:00 P.M., 2:00 A.M., 3:30 A.M., and 5:00 A.M. for administering medications, drawing blood samples, changing IV bags, and getting weigh-ins (to make sure that I was not retaining water, i.e., that my kidneys were working). Hard to feel rested and ready to be active after so many interruptions!

Despite these challenges, most of the patients on my floors did walk the hallways, dragging their IV poles with them. Oftentimes, if you started walking at the same time as someone else, either in the same direction, or in opposite directions, we would share a smile as we passed each other, but I never ended up walking with another patient, not even my roommates. While clearly some patients were too sick to manage these walks, the majority of patients on these floors were not bedridden. I am not sure to what degree this was a function of these particular floors—were the sicker, more advanced cancer patients treated on a different floor?

Since I wanted the staff to think of me as a "good patient," I took pride in my laps. The nursing and desk staff would encourage patients with cheerful comments each time they walked by the desk or nursing station. Nurses would also gently remind patients if they had not been out of their rooms for a while, encouraging them to take a walk.

It was uncomfortable, however, to keep passing other patients' rooms, especially if they had their doors opened. It felt voyeuristic to even glance in the room, but it was very hard not to since there was really no other place to look when walking the halls. Sometimes, patients would wave or smile as you walked past. Looking also gave you a peek into the world of other patients. As noted, patients often brought items from home to make their rooms more comfortable. One patient, a huge Eagles fan, hung a massive Eagles banner in his room, wore Eagles pajamas, and slept under an Eagles blanket. When passing his room, staff members and other patients could be heard saying, "Go Birds." Residents of the Philadelphia area will recognize that this phrase, which originally substituted for "Go Eagles," now functions as a way to greet fellow Philadelphians and folks from surrounding counties and wish them well.[36]

Walking with visitors made the task easier, less lonely, and less boring. When walking with my husband, children, or sister, we could talk about the world outside the hospital, stop by the communal kitchen to pick up a few items, and I could look at them, a lovely change from looking at the walls of the hallways and peeking into patient rooms. Talking also made time pass more quickly—what earlier had felt like drudgery now felt like a casual stroll.

Visitors provide many different roles in the hospital setting, some that can facilitate the smooth functioning of the floor, and others that might increase tensions between staff and the patient.[37] Recall my roommate's husband who slept in her bed, making it uncomfortable for nurses to come into the room at night. His sharing her bed created logistical challenges of accessing the patient for care—drawing blood, taking vitals, and so forth. But it also created an intimate scene that others did not want to disrupt. But visitors do help with simple tasks, such as getting water, adjusting pillows and blankets, and providing much needed distraction, company, and recreation.[38]

Nurses would also encourage all the patients I knew who were getting methotrexate to get up and get moving by reminding them that physical activity would help pass the drug and that as soon as it was in low-enough concentration in their blood sample, they could go home. This happy reminder helped me get moving a few times when the last thing I felt like doing was getting out of the bed.

Intimate Strangers

Assuming the sick role challenges the cloak of personal independence that Americans like to wear as members of this society. Illness can at least temporarily put us back into a situation of dependence, reminding us of our vulnerabilities, like when we were children. As we grow older and we are more likely to experience escalating morbidity, being increasing reliant on others can not only negatively influence our sense of self but also remind us too acutely of our mortality. Even mild illnesses remind us that we are indeed social animals, members of a wide community, and that we regularly rely on others, but a serious illness reminds us even more. We are not independent, despite how much we like to think that we are. In our complex society with extensive divisions of labor, daily I rely on countless people to sustain me. For example, despite how proud I am of the cucumbers and tomatoes that I harvest every summer from my garden, I purchase most of the calories that I need from local grocery stores and markets. I turn on my water tap and run the appliances in my house, often blissfully unaware of the many professionals behind the clean running water and the electricity streaming into my house, of the designers and builders of those appliances. And when an individual becomes seriously ill, they learn quite quickly that they need to rely on the expertise of the medical professionals to have a chance to survive the threat to their health.

Recognizing our crucial reliance on each other does not ultimately have to be an unpleasant experience. I have already written about the challenges associated with submitting to the expertise of the medical professional in my discussion of the doctor-patient relationship. Patients often find themselves having to submit to the touch and expertise of a professional who starts off at least as a stranger. Given the nature of the threat, the relationship between the medical professional and the patient, between patients, and between the patient and other ancillary personnel becomes what I define as one of "intimate strangers." In this chapter, I expand on this definition by using Georg Simmel's concept of the stranger and Lillian Rubin's concept of intimacy.[1,2] This unique relationship provides opportunities for types of intimacy in the face of mortality and existential threat that are not often expressed in our normal interactions with the numerous strangers we encounter in other institutional settings, where displays of our independence, functionality, and stoicism are highly valued and rewarded. Both Émile Durkheim and Georg Simmel discuss the need for indifference in most of our social interactions in order for us to survive the sheer number of encounters we experience in modern urban life.[1,3]

Simmel's Stranger

In his essay on "the stranger," Simmel describes a particular social category in society. Simmel defines the stranger as someone who physically is in the society and yet maintains social distance from the majority of the members of the group. Simmel's stranger is simultaneously part and not part of the society. With this definition, he differentiates the stranger from the outsider, one who has no connection at all to the group, and from the wanderer, someone transitory who will soon be leaving the physical and social space and therefore has no impetus for making connections with the group. Examples of Simmel's stranger include the "trader" and the "arbitrator." Because his stranger is "in" but not "of" the group, Simmel proposes that the stranger can occupy special roles. For example, the stranger is often accepted as a confidant, the receptacle of secrets, since they have enough knowledge about the group to understand the significance of the secret, but not enough power or connection to act upon the secret. This distinction is why they can also serve as judges and arbitrators—they have enough knowledge to understand the case, but they are impartial enough to rule fairly.

Patients as Strangers

The inpatient who spends any considerable time in the hospital shares some characteristics with Simmel's stranger. They are in the physical setting of the hospital, occupying the same space as the medical team, but they maintain a social distance (driven to a significant degree by differentials of education) that prevents them from ever being part of the "social" group of medical professionals.[4] They are not as transitory as the wanderer, as they are enmeshed in the setting for some time. They come into the setting with little power, but they are exposed to the literal life-and-death drama of the hospital.[5] They are given access to some of the "gritty knowledge" of the hospital experience, but they have no power or interest to act upon that knowledge, as they are primarily invested in their own interests (getting well), not in changing the culture or the institution.[6] On average, patients observe more of the institutional experience than do their visitors and interact more extensively with the medical team, developing a deep knowledge of the institution. But the patient also does not want to become a permanent member of the social group. Their transitory membership, however, gives them access to knowledge and secrets that people who have never been inpatients will not have, even if they spend their entire time in the institution avoiding the extensive experiential and therefore embodied knowledge that might warrant a permanent status.[7,8]

There are other enmeshed transitory populations. In my role as a professor, I often think about how my students are in transitory roles. While they are at the institution, we share physical spaces, and they get to see some of the gritty workings, but students' interest and investment in the university are significantly different than those of the professors or the administrators because the ideal is for them to leave after a specified time frame. We do not want students to obtain full membership in the social group, even if we do desire their loyalty once they graduate! (As the university sends donation requests to the graduate, so does the Abramson Cancer Center at Penn Medicine send funding requests to me.)

Rubin's Intimacy and the Patient–Medical Personnel Interaction

In her book *Intimate Strangers*, Rubin writes about the complex challenges men and women face when seeking intimacy in romantic relationships, but some of her discussions about intimacy extend to general human relationships. How and why do we seek intimacy? Here, I use some general concepts to explore intimate encounters in the medical setting.

Rubin defines intimacy as "some kind of reciprocal expression of feeling and though not out of fear or dependent need, but out of a wish to know another's inner life and to be able to share one's own."[2(p90)] She discusses how cultural conceptions about gender and wider institutional constraints can either enhance or impede our emotional lives, our ability to express and receive intimacy, noting that we still think of women as "more emotional" than men, and noting that in many occupational settings, displays of emotion and intimacy are discouraged in the name of productive functionality. How and why does the illness experience increase the need for intimacy, for patients and for medical personnel?

I propose that several factors increase the chances for more intimate interactions with relative strangers in medical settings. In adopting the sick role, the patient has already ideally placed significant trust in their medical professionals, allowing them access to their body in ways only allowed for select intimates outside the medical setting. The literal placing of their life in the hands of others is a physical and a cognitive act for the patient. The potential for intimate emotional encounters accompanies the permission for physical touch, though these must also be negotiated between patients and their caretakers.[9] And this potential in the inpatient setting extends to numerous people—not just doctors and nurses—as it truly is a team who is taking care of the patient, and a team whose members are regularly changing with each new shift. And this submission can displace some of the barriers to intimate encounters that might exist in other institutional settings, such as gender.

Another important factor is the mortal threat that serious illness presents. Recall that part of Rubin's definition of intimacy is a wish to be able to share one's inner life. When one's very existence is threatened, the desire to review and hopefully reclaim one's status in society markedly increases. In the hustle and bustle of our normative modern lives, we find little time for serious reflection. The serious threat to health is an opportunity to take stock of the life lived so far and to wish for the chance to experience what is still to come. When the future is threatened, cutting to the core of the meaning of the human experience takes on an urgency not present when we are healthy and preoccupied with fulfilling our normative roles. Opportunities for patients to share deeply personal and reflective thoughts can serve as incantations—prayers, even—hopefully heard by the universe.

As discussed in Chapter 8, sharing these thoughts might be quite important for the patient, but difficult for them to do with others, even their most significant others, since the conversation may scare the people with whom they share their life. To "be brave" for others requires in part not sharing some of the darkest and most fearful thoughts that cross patients' minds. Patients, however, may find willing ears among their medical team in the inpatient setting. I found many willing listeners during my inpatient stays—not with physicians, since their visits were typically quite limited, but with my nurses and other medical personnel. And, not surprisingly, these intimate encounters often occurred during physical interactions, when the medical professional was touching me in some significant way—accessing my port, changing intravenous medications, helping me into bed or into a wheelchair, and so forth. The close physical interaction sets the stage for a close emotional encounter. This experience is in some ways the pinnacle of a contradiction: You find yourself sharing some of the most profound experiences of your life with people whom you do not necessarily want to see again.

On the occasions when I shared intimate thoughts, fears, and so forth with someone, they inevitably shared some significant personal reflections or stories with me, making the exchange an intimate encounter. They shared stories that gave me a window into their "inner life." This sharing made the encounter feel complete and safe. I was not left merely sharing my fears or anxiety with a reluctant receptacle. The recipient acknowledged that they heard me by sharing some of their own internal life, demonstrating that they were a safe person and that they understood my need to be heard, to feel connected to the world. We connected when they also trusted me with their stories.

While some of these conversations were deeper and more intimate than I might even have had with a close friend, they were facilitated by the fact that these people, although professionals in a trusted institutional setting, were strangers. Ideally, once I completed my treatment, I would likely never see them again, or if I did, significant time would pass between our encounters, so, for example, I could share fears about my own mortality without thinking about how I would feel when we interacted next week—would I be self-conscious or feel vulnerable? Worried that they might think about me differently after I had shared such personal thoughts?

Their professional status also facilitated the exchanges, as I was confident that, given the nature of their work, none of my fears would surprise or upset them. Sharing your fear of dying with a nurse, who by the nature of their profession bears witness to life and death every day, is quite different than sharing that same fear with any nonmedical professionals or other strangers in your life, who might find the confessed fear shocking and distressing.

In addition to sharing intimate stories, some medical personnel also shared occupational "secrets" with me, an illustration of one of Simmel's proposed roles for the stranger. They shared challenges associated with their work, identifying me as a safe holder of these secrets.[10] I could appreciate these challenges, as I was bearing witness to them in real time, whether they be challenges associated with managing difficult patients or other challenges, such as being disrespected by a colleague. It seemed to provide them some comfort when, after they shared these secrets, I "saw" and validated the trials of their work. As a sociologist, I understand the power of being a participant observer in any setting. Sharing space, talking with, and carefully observing can provide insight into others' human experiences in deep, substantial ways.

However, I was also very aware that they were careful never to share secrets that could significantly upset me or that could only be shared with their medical colleagues. Many of us understand the need to vent about the challenges associated with our work. And the more stressful the work, the greater the need to vent to relieve built-up tension. But we also recognize that certain statements should be heard only by our colleagues and not by the people we serve. My fellow university instructors will often vent to each other about frustrating aspects of our students' behavior, but we are careful not to share these complaints in front of students. In our fiduciary roles, students need to trust that we genuinely care about them and will not abuse our positions of power, will not injure them. Hearing our gripes could lead them to worry that we will act upon these complaints in ways that might hurt them—for example, by grading them harshly.

The medical field is undeniably a high-pressure, high-tension profession, and venting by medical professionals is well documented. A classic example of professional venting in medical settings is the use of gallows humor. Katie Watson defines gallows humor as "humor that treats serious, frightening, or painful subject matter in a light or satirical way. Joking about death fits the term most literally, but making fun of life-threatening, disastrous, or terrifying situations fits the category as well."[11] Examples of gallows humor appear throughout Samuel Shem's classic book on the experience of medical residency, *The House of God*: "There is no body cavity that cannot be reached with a number fourteen needle and a good strong arm."[12] While this statement provides a humorous take on the challenges associated with providing medical care, the reference to aggressive force would be hard for any patient to hear and therefore is only "funny" to the medical professionals who might find themselves faced with this very challenge in their quest to help a patient. Therefore, medical professionals notoriously engage in gallows humor only out of the earshot of their patients, as part of their backstage interactions. Gallows humor and venting in general can help lighten situations that otherwise might feel overwhelming and tragic.[13,14] No stories or secrets shared with me by medical personnel were ever inappropriate for my "lay" patient ears.

Intimate Encounters

In previous chapters, I have shared descriptions of some of the intimate encounters I had with members of my nursing staff, so in this chapter, I focus on some encounters I had with nonmedical staff in the hospital setting. To protect workers' anonymity, I exclude some details about their personal characteristics that could reveal their identities. These stories come from my second inpatient stay, when I also had the tooth extraction, and I focus on the two patient escorts who took me to my dental appointments via wheelchair. The dental office was in a medical building across the street from the hospital.

As already shared, I was extremely uncomfortable while dealing with my dental emergency during my second inpatient stay. I was desperate to get some relief and have the tooth removed. As a reminder, there was some delay before I could get the tooth extracted, and I made two trips over to the dental office before I was finally able to get it removed.

During my first trip over, my escort was a lovely, gregarious middle-aged man with a hearty laugh. As we headed over to the building across the street, we engaged in normative small talk. As is common for this kind of small talk, he asked me where I was from and generally about how I was managing the treatments so far. Once he learned that I was a "local," from DELCO (Delaware County), we had a whole menu of topics we could chat about, as he was from DELCO too! Realizing how much pain I was in and how nauseated I was from the methotrexate infusion (and generally from my chemotherapy), he made an extra effort not to move me too quickly or change directions suddenly as he wheeled me through the various corridors so that we could cross over the bridge between the two medical buildings.

Once we got to the dental office, we quickly learned that there was no way that the dental staff could see me that afternoon. They were already too far behind schedule, and since I was an unexpected appointment—being "fit in" as an emergency—I would have to come back the next day. I was devastated, as I so desperately wanted some relief, but back to my room we would go. Already overwhelmed, exhausted, and in significant pain, despite my best efforts, I just started to cry.

Without skipping a beat, my escort took my hand and gave it a firm and comforting squeeze. I started to babble about how hard the whole experience was and how desperate I was for some relief. He said that he was so sorry, but he would get me back to my room and settled. He got me some tissues. Now behind me, ready to push me back to my room, he squeezed my shoulder and asked me if I was ready.

Diverting from normal small talk—DELCO, Go Birds!—he started asking me more personal questions. Did I have children? How old were they? Were they living in the area? What was I looking forward to once I finished treatment?

He had children too. He actually had a combined family, as he and his wife had their own children and they were raising her children from her first marriage—a big age range in the household, with older and younger children. And we talked and talked about the incredible privilege it is to be a parent. We also talked about the challenges, of the fantastic joys that are simultaneously mixed with heartaches. Of wanting to give them the world while also not spoiling them. Of finding it hard to find the words sometimes to describe that kind of love. And during the ride back to my room, I forgot about my pain and nausea as I allowed myself to be comforted and captivated by this poetic and intimate exchange of stories about parenting with my escort, a stranger whom I had known for less than one hour. He provided a level of care during this interaction that is unlikely a required part of his job description but that I still clearly value and honor.

During my second wheelchair trip, I had a different escort, a man who appeared to be in his early thirties. Like my first escort, he was very careful while pushing me through the halls. Since this trip was the next day, I was even more tired and irritable than I had been the day before. I had not slept well at all, and I felt depleted and defeated.

This man also engaged in normative small talk as we began our trip, and I apologized for not being a better conversationalist. He assured me that it was absolutely okay—he was there to take care of me!

When we got to the dental office, it was clear that they were running behind schedule yet again but that they would extract the tooth that day. I was relieved, but I was also in terrible pain, and it seemed unlikely that I was going to be able to get any additional morphine before the extraction. They told my escort to wheel me into a little bay with curtains where I could wait. He got me into the bay and then told me that he was going to wait with me for as long as possible before he had another escort assignment to keep me company until the dental staff could fit me in.

This simple recognition that I could use some company right then was such a great expression of care and kindness. I told him how much I appreciated his offer, but I did not want to get him in trouble with his dispatcher. He assured me that he would figure it out, not to worry. And he shared his view that sometimes patients needed more than just transportation. He told a story about recently waiting with a woman outside the hospital while she waited for her ride since she needed a little company. He felt that those extra moments were a vitally important part of his job.

And then we talked. He asked me to tell him about my non-patient life—was I married, did I have children, did I work? And I told him about my life beyond my current sick role. And I asked him about his life outside the hospital. And he told me about his teenage son, which made me gasp since he looked far too young to have a teenage son, and yes, he admitted, he was just a teenager himself when his girlfriend became pregnant. They tried to make a marriage work, but they were far too young, so they divorced within a few years. He worked hard to stay close to his son and worried about him all the time. He and his ex-wife had a good relationship and had done a pretty good job of co-parenting. I was honored to hear his stories.

Shortly after this conversation, I was taken to a treatment room, and blessedly, the tooth was extracted with relative ease, though not without significant pain. As they were getting me ready to send me back to my hospital room, I learned that my escort had managed to stay and would be taking me back! He had managed this, I learned, by ignoring one call from his dispatcher. I was so grateful, as I felt myself falling apart from the accumulated trauma, and having my new friend take me back was comforting. He carefully helped me back into the wheelchair, gave me comforting squeezes on my shoulder, and got me quickly back to my room.

Being an inpatient receiving chemotherapy and needing a tooth extraction offers few benefits, but experiences like these make the sick-role journey far less lonely and a bit more tolerable. I am forever grateful to all the intimate strangers I have encountered during my cancer experience.

The Last Infusion, Ringing the Bell, and Posttreatment Damage and Anxiety

As brutal as the treatment experience had been, I was terrified about what my experiences would be after treatment ended. Ideally, when we adopt the sick role, once we get better, we throw off the role and transition back to our pre-ill lives, but I was very aware of all the reasons why a simple return would not be possible. For one, the cancer experience is so extreme and brutal that one does not merely return to their pre-cancer life unchanged. The perilous treatment journey leaves physical and emotional scars. Another reason is the very nature of the beast. Because there is a risk of recurrence for all cancer patients, and because the medical team will not label a patient as cured until they remain cancer-free for at least five years posttreatment, even though active treatment has ended, I knew that I would still have one foot in the sick role and would not be able to fully dismiss its demands.

In this chapter, I use Arnold van Gennep's rites of passage analytical framework to explore the attempt to transition in and out of a cancer patient role, and I discuss some of the "rites" many cancer patients experience at the end of treatment.[1] Van Gennep's framework can help deepen our understanding of Talcott Parsons's sick role at all stages of the illness experience.

New Social Roles

During our lifespan, as we grow and age, we transition into new social roles. Societies define prescribed and desired roles for us to work toward. For example, the child ideally becomes an adult, and the student becomes a worker. Individuals might get married, become parents, and eventually become grandparents. Over time, the desirability and definition of these anticipated roles may change. Many roles also have biological and social elements. To help explore role transitions, let us consider what we mean by *adult*. From a biological standpoint, human communities have typically waited to define someone as an adult until they have completed puberty. But over the past 150 years, the average age of puberty for males and females combined has dropped from about sixteen years old to about twelve years old, due in part to better nutrition, but also as a result of environmental factors, such as exposure to chemicals and hormones used in food production.[2] In the United States, we generally do not legally consider someone an adult until they are eighteen years old, six years after they have obtained some adult biological capacity, the capacity for reproduction. By eighteen years old, the individual is deemed educated enough (having ideally finished high school by this age), and therefore mature enough, to make some legal judgments, such as getting married, signing contracts, and joining the military. But some of our legal definitions put even later dates on the achievement of "adult" status: twenty-one years old to consume alcohol and gamble, and in some states twenty-five years old to rent a car. So, in many modern societies, the transition from childhood to adulthood has numerous steps that consider a complex narrative of biological and social considerations. There is no one moment of transition from childhood to adulthood.

The transition from one role to another is typically celebrated through rituals, and these rituals are the subject of van Gennep's analytical framework. In his examination of rites of transition across many different human communities, he notes that they basically share three key stages: beginnings (rites of separation), middles (rites of liminality), and ends (rites of reaggregation).

As individuals prepare to move from one social role to the next, prescribed activities help communities collectively recognize the upcoming transformation. Take the example of marriage in some Western societies. The first stage involves the rites of separation, where the individuals to be married separate from their normal activities as they try on their anticipated new identities. Those getting married often are released from some normative obligations and responsibilities to prepare for the ritual, such as purchasing special outfits for the event, inviting those who will bear witness to the ritual, and even sometimes participating in body modifications, such as losing weight, getting new hairstyles, and/or seeking other cosmetic alternations, such as manicures and pedicures.

Van Gennep defines the liminal/middle stage as the point when transitioning individuals find themselves "betwixt and between" their old and new roles. During this stage, social norms are suspended. Van Gennep argues that this stage can be "dangerous," as people find themselves free from the expectations of their old social roles but bereft of the guidance of the new social roles. But he argues that this step is an important way to mark the separation of old and new roles. What are examples of this liminal stage when considering Western marriage rituals? Let us focus on the bachelor and bachelorette parties.

Prior to making the decision to get married, ideally, the two individuals are mature and stable enough to make this commitment to each other and enter a monogamous and enduring relationship. This hope suggests that the two have already demonstrated that they are functioning "adults" in society, having reached a status where they can materially and psychologically make this decision. No longer will they behave as "single" people, seeking the romantic attention of others. But during the bachelor/bachelorette party, social norms of "good behavior" are suspended, and participants may engage in behavior that is likely to be permanently prohibited once the individual accepts the new social role. In the United States, these behaviors include the consumption of considerable amounts of alcohol, playful encounters with people to whom the about-to-be married people might be sexually attracted, and other rowdy behaviors.[3] These parties can be "dangerous," as they may lead people to realize that they are not ready to complete the transition to the new role.

The final stage is reaggregation or reincorporation, when a final ritual confirms the new status of the individual and introduces them to society in their new social role. The final stage in this example is the formal wedding ceremony. When the ceremony begins, the two individuals are still "single." After their participation in the exchange of vows of commitment and often the exchange of rings, they are then introduced to the wedding guests as a married couple.

Rites of Passage and the Cancer Sick Role

I have already reviewed elements of the transition to the sick role for cancer patients in previous chapters, including, according to van Gennep's framework, what we might call the first stage, the rite of separation from the "healthy" role—the at-least-partial departure from normal roles and responsibilities as a consequence of the illness. Patients cannot fulfill all their normal social roles since they are physically incapacitated and need to devote some time and energy to getting medical treatment. We could argue that the separation stage for the cancer patient also includes their physical transformation once they begin treatment, in particular the separation of the patient from aspects of their pre-cancer appearance; the loss of hair is one of the most noticeable, but as noted earlier, differences may also include extreme fatigue, weight loss or gain, and changes in skin and nails. It is important to remember that this separation stage can be quite traumatic, as an individual's fulfillment of normative roles and physical presentation of self might be essential elements of their identity.

The liminal stage for the cancer patient is during treatment, when the patient finds themselves "betwixt and between" their pre- and post-cancer treatment selves. As previously noted, van Gennep considers this time dangerous, when the individual is unmoored from aspects of their previous social role and not yet connected to their new role (in this case, hopefully as a "cancer survivor"). For the cancer patient, this danger is underscored by their literally being between life and possible death. If the patient cannot survive treatment, the liminal period, they are unlikely to survive at all. And I have discussed ways in which cancer patients try to survive this dangerous period—staying connected to some aspects of their pretreatment life, trying to maximize behaviors that might help them survive, and often participating in some comforting rituals, such as donning favorite lucky socks on treatment day. But during the treatment stage, patients are also permitted to engage in behaviors that otherwise would not be acceptable and signal the danger they are in: taking naps due to extreme fatigue, vomiting and/or not enjoying or tolerating certain foods, and expressing being overwhelmed by their illness status. They are also released from some norms of the public presentation of self.

The patient and others around them can find themselves sharing aspects of this liminal stage. Since others are also unsure whether the patient will survive this dangerous time and since the patient has already been released from some of their normative responsibilities, some relationships may be temporarily renegotiated or revised. The ill worker may not be able to fulfill their duties at work, but colleagues might be hesitant to replace them while they are undergoing treatment in case they come back. Spouses ideally will not seek to replace their ill spouse, but their relationship may significantly change in terms of daily household management; more poignantly, their habits of intimacy may change. Children may find themselves caring for their ill parent. And all people within the cancer patient's inner circles may find themselves mourning the potential loss of a person with whom they were making future plans.

One Day at a Time

Another common piece of advice given to cancer patients during the treatment stage is to adopt a "one day at a time" attitude. Since the journey through treatment may be so long that the end is hard to see (and possibly unreachable), this advice is given to help the patient direct their attention to the immediate experience of living and not spend time fretting about the future. As stated on a Mayo Clinic website: "Take one day at a time. It's easy to forget to do this during stressful times. When the future is not sure, organizing and planning may suddenly seem like too much work."[4] It may seem like too much work, but more heartbreakingly, thinking about the future may also give rise to sorrow. While I was undergoing treatment, my eldest was planning their wedding, and my son was applying to medical school. If I let my thoughts drift too far into the future, I imagined the possibility of not attending the wedding and not attending the white-coat ceremony. These thoughts left me bereft.

The "one day at a time" perspective also allows patients to avoid dwelling on the fact that the very challenging side effects from treatment will either persist or get worse. The fatigue will accumulate, the nausea will get more severe, and the collective injury will be felt. If the patient focuses a bit too long on that reality, the courage to get in the car and head in for an infusion may disappear. As my treatment progressed, I would frequently sob before taking the deepest breath I could, collecting my items, and heading in for my next infusion. As I said to my head infusion nurse during my last outpatient infusion, the novelty of the experience, which was at least a distraction for a while, had completely worn off by the tenth session.

The Hero's Journey and Reintegration

In addition to van Gennep's rites of passage framework, a review of the narrative archetype, the "hero's journey," can give insight into the cancer patient's experience of trying to navigate their illness. This narrative form involves a hero who goes on an adventure, learns a lesson, wins a victory with newfound knowledge, and then returns home, transformed.[5] The hero's journey is typically defined by three essential steps:[6]

- **The departure:** The hero leaves the familiar world behind.
- **The initiation:** The hero learns how to navigate this unfamiliar world.

- **The return:** The hero returns to their familiar world but has been changed by the experience.

Some popular examples of hero's journeys include the Harry Potter series, the Star Wars saga, *The Lion King*, *The Wizard of Oz*, and *The Lord of the Rings*.[7]

The Cancer Patient's Hero's Journey

The cancer patient's official departure begins with the diagnosis. But as discussed in Chapters 1 and 2, diagnosis can take a significant amount of time—on average, about five months.[8] Given the demands of the diagnostic process, even before a cancer diagnosis is confirmed, the individual has already begun departing from their familiar world. Another common feature of the hero's journey is that the hero is often unsure about following their call to adventure, not unlike the patient's hesitation to accept the sick role. In a classic hero's tale, often a mentor figure convinces the reluctant hero to accept the adventure. For the cancer patient, these mentors can be concerned family members and medical professionals.

Once the diagnosis is confirmed, the patient often quickly enters a new unfamiliar world, where they must learn how to navigate new doctors, new offices, and strange medical procedures. As noted in Chapter 2, this experience often involves the literal navigation of a world of new medical buildings and offices. I was overwhelmed at first when navigating the new floors and hallways of the Abramson Cancer Center and HUP. Where were the elevators, the bathrooms, the infusion center, the X-ray area, the parking garage, and so forth? As noted earlier, on my journey into this new world, I was guided by any number of very kind concierges.

During the initiation, the hero, now in the new world, must face a series of challenging tasks to overcome some obstacle or enemy. The hero must use everything they have been learning on the journey to succeed. The cancer patient facing any of and all the classic treatment protocols—surgery, chemotherapy, radiation therapy, and/or immunology—surely faces a series of very challenging tasks that test every ounce of perseverance that they can muster. The patient is also required to employ the new skills acquired during the initiation—how to manage significant side effects and still keep accepting and completing the tasks. The prize for completing all the tasks is hopefully getting into remission, but we also often anticipate that the patient, like the hero, has also gained some wisdom from the experience. What special message or insight from this experience does everyone expect the hero to share?

The Return and the "Survivor" Label

In a classic hero's journey, the hero, having completed all their tasks, is ready to return to their world. But in the classic tale, the hero recognizes that they have completed a "personal metamorphosis" and have been changed.[6] For cancer patients, the return begins at the end of active treatment, but the return can be a terrifying time, as the patient must navigate the liminal state between stopping treatment and achieving the label of "cured" without the direct regular support of their oncology team. And they then begin to assess the ways in which they have changed.

In earlier chapters, I discussed some of the challenges of using warrior metaphors for patients' illness experiences. One of my motivations for using the hero's journey here as an analytical framework is that once treatment has ended, the cancer warrior becomes the cancer "survivor," the hero of their own story. But similar to the problems associated with the warrior metaphor, challenges and burdens can be associated with donning the survivor metaphor posttreatment.

One challenge is the extreme length of the "posttreatment to cure" phase—typically about five years. It is problematic for cancer patients to adopt the survivor label when they do not know whether they will survive until they have reached the five-year posttreatment anniversary without a recurrence. Prematurely donning the label is also a fear—could I jinx my own chances of surviving if my hubris tempts me to accept the label before I have finished my journey?

Another challenge is patients' inability to fully relinquish the sick role since during these five years posttreatment, they are still participating in medically related tasks, such as scans and follow-up visits. Each follow-up visit, each test, is a rough reminder that the patient is not yet out of danger.[9] But because they are no longer in active treatment, others in their social and occupational circles are less tolerant of the former patient's adoption of sick-role behaviors. Many are eager for the patient to joyfully embrace the survivor label and the obligations that come with it.

So, what is a survivor? Kris Carr provides this definition of the cancer survivor: "A survivor is a triumphant person who lives with, after, or in spite of a diagnosis or traumatic event. Survivors refuse to assume the identity of their adversity. They are not imprisoned by the constructs of a label. Instead, survivors use their brush with mortality as a catalyst for creating a better self. We transform our experience in order to further evolve spiritually, emotionally, physically, and mentally."[10]

Researchers and cultural analysts have noted that central to the cancer survivor identity is the idea that cancer creates a "better self." The traumatic experience provides opportunities for personal growth and a chance for a "makeover."[11,12,13] Even medical practitioners see a cancer diagnosis as an opportunity for patients to transform their lives, recognize their past mistakes, and adopt more health-promoting behaviors—in short, it is a teachable moment.[14] This focus on hopeful individual transformation reflects core elements of popular American and medical culture and reflects aspects of the hero's journey and our desire to interpret trauma as redemptive and ultimately positive.[15]

In fact, one of the obligations of the cancer-survivor label is to demonstratively express gratitude and joy from a deeper appreciation of life. Generalized others are happy to bestow the survivor label and celebrate the post-cancer identity, but they are far less willing to accept accounts of how brutal the experience was. As Judy Segal notes in her newspaper editorial, "Cancer Isn't the Best Thing That Ever Happened to Me," these survivor narratives have coercive aspects: "If, as a person with cancer, you violate the code of optimism, or if cancer somehow failed to improve you, you'd better be quiet."[16] Medical professionals also expect displays of gratitude. During my third posttreatment appointment with my oncologist—so nine months posttreatment—I was feeling emotionally overwhelmed. I shared with him that I was getting support from a therapist, but since stopping cancer treatment, I was beginning to fully realize how brutal the experience had been and how difficult it is while in active treatment to acknowledge just how hard it is. As noted earlier, unchecked recognition would make it very hard to get in the car to go to your appointment. In a rare moment of demonstrating a terrible bedside manner, he impatiently asked me whether I had tried "practicing gratitude." Remember, I was not asking him for help—I had already informed him that I was getting support from my therapist. He went on to suggest that I think about all the patients who had been diagnosed since the COVID pandemic had begun and what a hard experience they were having. I was momentarily speechless. And then I shared with him the words of my dear friend who had knitted my lovely blue hat: "Trauma and brutality are not competitions that I am trying to win." And as my therapist often reminded me, just because an individual does not have the most objectively brutal life imaginable does not mean that their suffering has no legitimacy. Ideally, we are all working to reduce human suffering. And ideally, we can allow people to give voice to their suffering. Instead, we paradoxically hold people who have been brutalized by their illness experience to an expectation of creating a better self, and we silence their authentic narratives.

The burden of being a better self, the survivor, the role model, was discussed by the families of the pediatric cancer patients I interviewed in the late 1980s. Whenever they went back to the Children's Hospital of Pennsylvania for checkups, the "survivors" would be paraded around the department for all to see. Thirty-five years ago, remission rates for pediatric cancer were not as good as they are now, so these children were examples of treatments that had worked. The parents and the children talked about the burden that came with the magical thinking that there must be some important reason why these children had survived when other children had not. People had great expectations for what these surviving children would achieve. But many of the parents noted that the treatments had negatively affected their children. One set of parents reported that the radiation therapy that their child diagnosed with a brain tumor had received had decreased his IQ, a side effect that still exists today, despite better, less destructive treatment protocols.[17] They believed that it was unfair to have such great expectations for their son since he now struggled in school. The collective hope that the survivor will somehow "give back" to the world as a tribute to their good fortune, will fulfill some destiny, is a tough standard to hold the hero to since they likely have been damaged during their journey.

I am not arguing that donning the survivor label and expressing gratitude do not have some positive functions for the cancer patient posttreatment. Every person needs hope, and I was extremely grateful that I appeared to be in remission when I was released from treatment. I joyfully embraced the thought that I would attend my eldest's wedding and that I would get to attend my son's white-coat ceremony. But I would argue that wider acceptance of the very complex cancer-patient narrative is important for every cancer patient and survivor.

Arthur Frank also argues for wider appreciation of and attention to patients' narratives in his work *The Wounded Storyteller*.[18] Sharing some features similar to the hero's journey framework, he describes three types of patient narratives among his research participants—stories of restitution, chaos, and quest. Restitution stories focus on the anticipation of getting well. In chaos narratives, illness is experienced with seemingly no end and no redeeming outcomes. In quest narratives, patients find that their illness experiences can help them transform their lives. But in all three cases, Frank argues, patients' narratives become public testimonies that reveal core truths about the human condition and shared human experiences. I agree with Frank that we need to provide more ways to listen to the complex and sometimes-fraught patient narratives, accepting testimonies of the good and the bad, the chaotic and redemptive, to fully appreciate authentic narratives.

The Last Infusion: Ringing the Bell

At the end of my last infusion, I was invited to "ring the bell." The ringing of a bell has become a national ritual in cancer treatment centers to mark the end of treatment: "For patients with cancer and their healthcare team, the 'ringing of the bell' is a significant moment—a point in time that signals the end of active treatment."[19]

As a sociologist, I thought this ritual curious in part because people on the infusion floor may be in a variety of different stages of their care. Some are just beginning the journey. Some are nearing the end. Some may be facing the challenge of a recurrence—they may have rung the bell before, but now they are back in treatment. And some may never ring the bell. During my months of treatment, most ringers showed some restraint. The ringing could be heard on the entire floor, but it was not boastful. This discretion may be part of the culture of HUP, but I also suspect that most "ringers" are aware of the variety of stages represented on the floor and therefore show some restraint. Hearing the bell during my early infusions gave me hope, as I suspect that it did for everyone on the floor—that there might be an end, that the act of willingly poisoning our own bodies would actually save our lives. When it was my turn, my head nurse that day recited a short poem, and then I gave the bell one ring. As I had done when others had rung the bell during my infusion, patients in the infusion rooms up and down the hallway clapped. The patient and the support person in the room right next to the bell came to their door and congratulated me. This shared experience reminded us all that we are members of a club that we never wanted to join, but the support that strangers sharing a life experience can provide to each other during these times—the knowing nod, the smile as they pass each other in the hallway—is extremely important. Patients cannot but feel less alone on the journey during these shared moments.

The Last Scan and Release Instructions

During the first few weeks after my last PET scan, I experienced extreme anxiety. Having studied the cancer experience, I was not surprised. While being released from treatment is celebrated, it also feels a bit like being pushed off a cliff. I was thrilled that the PET scan "look[ed] clear," but my doctors and I knew that there still might be some cancer cells hiding in my body. As horrible as I had felt during treatment, I had taken some comfort in knowing that I was doing something active to address the problem. And I wanted to know what I could do now.

Recall that I maintained as many of my pre-cancer healthy lifestyle behaviors as possible during treatment to try to maximize my chance of achieving remission. I had every intention of continuing them posttreatment, even though by this point, I was quite fatigued. But as had been true throughout my experience, I had no idea what had caused me to develop primary bone lymphoma, so I could not actively avoid potential triggers or adopt any additional behaviors that might help prevent a recurrence. But the survivor's expectation was that I would actively work (as a result of becoming a "better self," appreciating life, and having benefitted from teachable moments) to accept my responsibility for managing the risk of recurrence.[13] The danger of a hyper-focus on the worthy transformative nature of a cancer experience and the narrow focus on the individual's responsibility to better themselves, their health habits, and avoid recurrence draw attention away from the environmental factors outside our control that contribute to the development of cancer for all of us.

When I shared these anxieties with my oncologist, he acknowledged that my situation was very challenging. He went on to say that it might also be more challenging for me since at the time of my diagnosis, I had not had classic lymphoma symptoms, such as night sweats and enlarged lymph glands, so there might not be obvious signs of recurrence. After seeing my face drop, he quickly followed up with "Well, certainly, don't play with Roundup!" (the active ingredient in the weed killer has been linked to an increased risk of non-Hodgkin's lymphoma as well as other cancers, such as lymphocytic leukemia[20]). As an avid organic gardener, I never played with Roundup and would certainly not start now! He then emphatically said, "Well, just go out there and live your life," while quickly following up with "But let me know immediately if something doesn't feel right." At this point in the experience, hardly anything about my body felt right. I was bald, constantly nauseated, and extremely fatigued. But I understood what he was trying to tell me.

Assessing My Damage and Managing My Fear of Recurrence

My assessment of my damage began shortly after I was released from treatment. During treatment, focusing on "one day at a time" left little space to think about the damage, to think about how my body might be permanently changed by this illness journey. Would my hair grow back? Would it be the same or different? Would I be able to play soccer again, and squash? Would I regain the strength in my right arm? How long would it take to assess which impairments were temporary and which were permanent?

I was unnerved after my first physical therapy appointment just weeks posttreatment to assess my right arm and shoulder, and to also assess my core and leg strength. For the first time in my life, my left arm was evaluated as stronger, more mobile, and more stable than my right. As my therapist put me through my paces, I almost cried, as I could not keep my right arm stable. It kept shaking as she asked me to hold it in various positions and to resist her movement of my arm. I was so upset because I did not really know how bad my right arm and shoulder were until then. And I was sad, not because I did not think that I would be able to regain a lot of strength and mobility with her help but because it was my right arm. As noted before, I am right-handed, and my right arm is the way I most fully have interacted with and manipulated my world. It is primarily with my right arm that I write, cook, shake hands, garden, and so forth. I realized that this vital extension of myself had been damaged.

Some of the damage I felt also ignited my fear that the cancer was recurring. Every time I felt a twinge in my arm, or my leg, or my pelvis, it was hard not to feel the fear rise in my throat, especially since pain had been my primary symptom. Was it back? My physical therapist was able to help me interpret some of the particular pains I was experiencing based on our exercises, and that helped me take a few breaths and reset my psyche. But I was also instructed by my oncologist and my physical therapist to keep a journal noting when I had pain and discomfort and to keep track of the location of the pain, when I first noticed the discomfort, and whether it was getting better or worse.

The level of fear I felt in these early weeks and months was, frankly, debilitating. I found it nearly impossible to get back to "living my life" when I felt derailed by even the most minor aches and pains. But living at a stage of such heightened anxiety is simply not sustainable. You must learn to let the fear go in bits, and with each passing week, it did start to get a little easier. I understood that for the rest of my life, I would be more vigilant. But I also hoped that with each week and month, with each step closer to the magical five-year mark, the vigilance would not feel so heavy. I came to accept that the fear would never fully go away, but I tried not to feed it. And as my hair started to regrow, and the nausea started to subside, I celebrated the body that was no longer having to manage infusions of antibodies and poisons, and I started to walk a little faster and even jog a bit.

Continuing the Assessment

At my first three-month follow-up visit with my oncologist, I was reminded of some of the potential long-term damage that could result from my treatment with R-CHOP, a primary one being cardiotoxicity (heart damage).[21] My doctor noted that if there was damage, it would not be reversible through lifestyle habits since it had been caused by treatment with anthracyclines, but it also might not show up for ten years. I could not completely "healthy lifestyle" my way out of the damage, though resuming as healthy a lifestyle as possible would clearly help me manage it. Since I learned this news only three months out of treatment, I experienced the reminder like a kick in the gut. I had been aware when I started treatment that it might cause permanent damage, but I had also known that I would die without it. I had made a short-term decision to try to survive, understanding that I might have to pay the devil later. I suspected that I did have some heart damage. I often woke up in the middle of the night with palpitations, which, oddly, I could hear most loudly when I was lying on my left side, so to fall back to sleep, I had to turn over on my right. I had an echocardiogram when I got close to my five-year posttreatment anniversary to assess where I stood; it showed some damage since the first echocardiogram, but nothing worrisome at this point.

A few months posttreatment, I developed chronic tendonitis in my left foot. That finally settled down after a few months of physical therapy, but what has remained in that same foot is significant sensory neuropathy. It is difficult to explain to someone who never has experienced neuropathy the dual sensation of a loss of feeling (numbness and diminished awareness) coupled with periodic prickling and tingling, burning, and sharpness.[22] The greatest challenge from the neuropathy is walking down a slope or walking downstairs. Because of the diminished sensation, I am often unsure of whether my left foot has properly landed on whatever surface I am traipsing on. Even when I am directly looking at where I am stepping, my visual assessment does not match my body's sensation, and on more than one occasion, my failure to feel where my foot has landed has resulted in my falling. This reason is why I am extra-vigilant when going downstairs. I hold onto the rail quite tightly, making sure that I am not carrying anything in one hand. I have more than once fallen on hiking trails when I have been out with my dogs since there are no handrails in nature! I have stepped down, failed to coordinate my visual and physical messages, and crumpled to the forest floor. While my dogs have patiently waited for me to get back up, I have reminded them of how lucky they are to have four feet!

In addition to the neuropathy, four years posttreatment, I still experience significant unexpected and sudden cramping in all my limbs, coupled with periodic episodes of trigger fingers and trigger toes. Anyone who has ever experienced a charley horse, a muscle cramp that can last from seconds to minutes, knows how painful it can be! Although harmless, the sensation is incredibly uncomfortable. Although this side effect from cancer and its treatments are well documented online, my cancer team was hesitant to acknowledge my experiences and had no clear recommendation for me on how to manage the cramping.[23,24] While it was suggested by my oncologist and my physical therapist that perhaps I was dehydrated or that my magnesium or potassium levels were low, none of my blood work has ever suggested that these issues were contributing factors. I tried supplements for a while with no change in frequency or duration of cramping, so now I approach each episode with some focused breathing. I found that trying to stretch the cramping muscle during an active episode increased the pain and duration.

The episodes of trigger finger and trigger toe are also quite painful and have occurred at unusual times. For example, I often experience trigger finger after writing on the chalkboard in a classroom on the Moravian University campus. I find myself unable to move my fingers—most frequently, my index finger—and remove the chalk. I then inform the students that I need a minute before I can resume teaching! Since I am often teaching medically related sociology classes, these moments can lead to instruction about a concept, and thankfully, a chance for us to laugh together.

While my hair did return, it never returned to its pretreatment fullness and thickness. I now have a quite noticeable "thinned" spot on the top of my head, which I can hide to some degree by twisting my hair up. My eyelashes have also not fully returned. They remain ghosts of their former selves. My eyelashes are now so thin, I have often contemplated wearing fake lashes.

The frequent and unpredictable cramping and the sensory neuropathy have significantly affected my posttreatment life. It appears at this point that I have permanently lost some function in my hands and feet. In addition to these unwanted side effects, I continue to experience significant fatigue. I have described this state as feeling beaten up by my cancer experience, a sense that the winds have gone out of my sails. The lingering fatigue coupled with the restrictions of the COVID-19 pandemic made it difficult to fully celebrate achieving remission by completing some bucket-list items, such as traveling, starting a new hobby, buying land so I could start a dog rescue organization, and so forth. I regularly feel tension between fulfilling my duty as the returned hero, the cancer survivor, by living life to its fullest when I am also living life as a very tired sensory-impaired individual who wants to take a nap.

Continued Reintegration

Parsons's sick role anticipates that the patient will return to their pre-illness life, but in the case of cancer, the cancer-survivor model is more closely related to van Gennep's rite of transition to a different state—ideally as a new, better, more enriched human being, but also potentially as a damaged hero. It may take many months or years for the cancer patient to fully reintegrate, and during those years of reflection, they may make decisions about new ways of living in the world, perhaps due to new physical limitations, and perhaps in recognition of the shortcomings of their pre-cancer lives.[25] Many cancer survivors note that many details about their lives may change while they were in treatment. Workplace compositions may change. Family and friends may transition to new stages of their lives. Holiday celebrations may happen that the patient cannot attend. Time marches on while the patient is on their journey.

Studies have shown that some cancer survivors discontinue some of their pre-cancer activities to avoid having to face the damage resulting from their cancer experience.[24] Even four years later, I have not played soccer, as I feel ill-equipped to run up and down the field, controlling the ball with my sensory-deprived feet! But I have not even tried, and that is how I recognize that I am avoiding facing the possibility that I could not do it. I can happily report, however, that I have taken up pickleball, and I adore the sport.

We can understand why many social institutions want the cancer patient in remission to return to normal as quickly as possible. Employers are likely anxious for the employee to resume their pre-cancer workload. And family and friends are likely anxious to celebrate the patient's new status—in remission—and hopefully restore their normal relationships, especially those closest to the patient, who may have invested significantly in their care during treatment and may themselves be drained from the experience. But if most of the people around the patient desire a quick return to normalcy, where will patients find others who will acknowledge that the journey is not over, that the process of reintegration is demanding and long? When I am released from treatment, if I no longer can lay claim to the rights of the sick role—in particular, the release from some normal obligations—and if the cancer-survivor label demands a sunny and grateful disposition, then who hears and acknowledges the challenges of this new stage of the experience, betwixt and between active treatment and the magical five-year mark? I address this question in the next chapter.

Belonging to a Club You
Never Wanted to Join

A Virtual Support Community

In his 1972 article, "Insiders and Outsiders: A Chapter in the Sociology of Knowledge," Robert K. Merton discusses the theoretical limits of fully, authentically understanding human experiences outside our own personal experiences, despite scholars in the discipline of sociology striving for as full as possible an understanding of this diverse collectivity as a core intellectual pursuit.[1] He notes that for us to get as close as possible to this understanding requires great trust in and acceptance of the knowledge and perspectives shared by others. Under conditions where this trust breaks down, groups may start to claim special access to particular kinds of knowledge and perspectives—that is, "insider" knowledge—that by definition cannot be accessed by "outsiders." Within the discipline at the time he wrote the article, he notes that arguments were being made that only Black scholars could understand the Black experience and, likewise, that only White scholars could fully understand the White experience. Once extreme claims like these were legitimized, Merton warns, it would soon follow that only men could understand men and women understand women. This line of thinking taken to the extreme would end with only each individual capable of fully understanding themselves, a tragic conclusion for a discipline that attempts to create comprehensive understanding and appreciation of the human condition.

Merton acknowledges that some fools were "given to quick and superficial forays into the group or culture under study" and therefore would always remain outsiders, but he fears that the insider doctrine went beyond this carelessness. He worries that the argument claimed that even the most careful and sincere outsider could never comprehend the other since they had not been socialized into the group or collected the same experiences, and therefore they could never acquire the necessary "intuitive sensitivity."

While Merton laments the limits an insider/outsider perspective presented for the discipline of sociology, a limitation on people who were intentionally and earnestly striving to understand the experiences and perceptions of people like and unlike them, the insider and outsider framework can help us explore interactions between people who would like to remain outsiders, not fully understanding others' experiences, and the insiders who might be striving to influence the public collective understanding of their reality. I have already addressed some of this public conflict in my discussions of the demands of the sick role, of the cancer warrior metaphor, and of being a cancer survivor. Is there a collective reluctance to understand cancer patients' experiences as fully as possible, in part because of the brutality of those experiences? Do outsiders blissfully want to remain outsiders, leaving insiders—cancer patients—seeking other insiders who share lived access to knowledge about their experiences with cancer and can help validate them? And how does this collective group of cancer insiders work to influence the public understanding of their experiences?

As noted in Chapter 12, the process of reintegration for the cancer patient can take years as the patient in remission navigates the magical five years posttreatment, and yet this navigation must be done after the patient has lost certain rights that came with their sick role—in particular, the right to express fear. They also lose their regular access to their oncology team and regular access to other patients. They celebrate giving up the burden and demands of treatment, but they find themselves neither in the land of the sick nor in the land of the well. The patient in remission but stuck in the five-year posttreatment phase of treatment-free periodic checks and appointments becomes an example of Everett V. Stonequist's marginal human.[2] Having left the precancer world of the healthy but finding that they cannot yet successfully reintegrate into that life (since these frequent checkups remind the patient that they are not out of danger), the patient during this time finds themselves straddling the margin of two worlds, a full member of neither.

Seeking Support and Finding a Community

As noted earlier, being released from active treatment left me feeling adrift, no longer comforted by my active participation in my treatment, but still unsure whether I would remain in remission. The expectation, however, was that I would resume all my pre-cancer roles with their corresponding responsibilities and "live my life." My therapist suggested that I join a cancer support group to help deal with this unease of living betwixt and between my pre- and post-cancer lives, but it was hard to carve out the time to research the availability of a group and commit to joining, given the resumption of all my pre-cancer obligations! And then I found a very important community of insiders, @Thanks-Cancer on Twitter (now X). Despite the fact that members of this extensive online community (sixteen thousand-plus members) have experienced or are experiencing a vast array of different types of cancers, we have discovered far more commonalities than differences. We have a place where we can share our cancer narratives freely, without rejection or judgment from outsiders who are unwilling and/or unable to sit in the angst and fear that cancer patients face. In this community, patients can be unconstrained by the demands of being a good patient, a brave warrior, a grateful survivor. We hold each other when others are too scared to do so. We post pictures of waiting-room or infusion-day feet, of bald heads and scars, without fears of negative comments or expressions of impatience from family, friends, and coworkers who no longer want to think about our cancer experiences. We confess our scan anxiety, knowing that our fellow insiders can comfort us through the simple acknowledgment that they know firsthand this feeling. No one tries to console the anxious poster by saying that everything will be okay since every community member knows that it might not be—there are no guarantees—but we can assure each other that we in fact do understand and are ready to listen and send support.

Insiders as Intimate Strangers

In Chapter 11, I described some of the intimate encounters that happen between patients and between patients and their medical team during treatment. In this chapter, I talk more about the intimacy that develops between cancer patients.

The pre-cancer experiences of the patients being treated in one oncology department are incredibly rich and varied, but by some stroke of fate, all the patients end up together at a particular time in a particular department. A common shared experience is that of having a pre-cancer and hopefully "healthy" past. They are now bound together by sharing the same waiting rooms and walking the same hallways of the inpatient floors. And if someone joins an online community, the members of the community are bound by the shared experience of either currently going through or having been through cancer treatment. Despite the heterogeneity of their pre-cancer lives, the demands of being a cancer patient create new bonds, a new intimate kinship.

Photos of "waiting-room feet," a picture taken by the patient of their calves and feet from their first-person perspective as they are sitting in a waiting room, are a familiar picture to any patient who also spent or is spending what feels like countless hours waiting for tests, appointments, scans, or infusions. And photographs of bald heads or surgery scars remind viewers where they have been and help prepare the newly diagnosed for what might be coming. These selfies and pictures are not the perfect versions we feel compelled to post on social media sites to illustrate our nearly perfect happy lives, our airbrushed and well-coiffed selves. These raw pictures produce an intimacy among the viewers, strangers though they may be beyond their shared experience of cancer and now of following an online community.[3] Those feet could very well be my feet. Those scars look exactly like my scars. There are others like me. The company the shared narratives and photographs provide is highly comforting. You cannot help feeling less alone.

Unmet Needs

Current and former cancer patients seek each other out during and after treatment to help fill unmet needs. Reviews of studies on patients' unmet needs found that 34% of survivors report having more than five moderate or severe unmet needs at the beginning of the posttreatment phase, and for many of these patients, these needs remained unmet even six months later.[4] Another review of fifty-seven studies quantified the unmet needs of survivors and found that as many as 83% have experienced unmet informational needs during the posttreatment period.[5] Patients reported needing information and support regarding physical concerns, activities of daily living, supportive care, sexuality, communication, psychosocial matters, and finances. But oncology teams are not generally well equipped to provide systematic guidance and support to patients once they end treatment. But current and former patients can be wells of information!

Friendship Based on Strangership

I have found it poignant that I have come to care so much about "strangers," albeit "insiders," across America and across the globe through @ThanksCancer. In Chapter 11, I used Georg Simmel's definition of the stranger to talk about the position of the patient in the hospital, bearing witness to the drama but having no plans to become a permanent member. In his work *Modernity and Ambivalence*, Zygmunt Bauman comes to define the stranger as someone who is present yet unfamiliar, someone having the potential of being intriguing and compelling but also having the potential of being uncontrollable and therefore threatening.[6] Springboarding off Simmel's, Bauman's, and others' musings on the definition of *stranger*, Mervyn Horgan defines *strangership* to focus on what characterizes the relationship between strangers rather than what divides them.[7] For Horgan, strangership is based on sharing the most general characteristics, even as broad as being present in the same place at the same time. If more characteristics are shared or become increasingly shared over time, people transition from being "strangers" to being "intimates." But Bauman and Horgan do not think that experiences between strangers, or a strangership, are by design insubstantial social bonds. Rather, they argue, whatever becomes the basis for the shared experience between strangers (even if merely being present at the same place at the same time) could expand our moral capacities by creating some measure of social solidarity among heterogeneous societies or groups. By this argument, experiencing cancer and becoming a member of a cancer support community can expand our moral capacities by creating social solidarity and intimacy between strangers.[3,6]

The variety of cancers represented among an online community such as @ThanksCancer is vast, and therefore so is the assortment of treatment protocols. This trait differs from groups that form based on common cancers, such as groups limited to breast-cancer or lung-cancer patients. Given the variety of protocols, chemotherapy drugs vary, as do some of the side effects. Some patients also experience surgery and radiotherapy. But in this forum, maintaining solidarity eclipses the diverse details, and no one argues that their experience is harder or worse than others'. Fears, anxiety, tips on navigating the worst side effects, good news, bad news, and gallows humor are all shared in ways that challenge the norm of polite conversation between strangers. Intimate revelations about how bad someone feels or how scared someone is are honestly and blatantly professed in ways we would not so directly share with even the most intimate people in our lives. We talk about our nausea, diarrhea, constipation, extreme fatigue, and drainage sites from surgery without worrying that the reader will be squeamish. The freedom to have impolite conversations adds to the creation and maintenance of this intimate solidarity between strangers, a solidarity that does not require common background, location, socioeconomic status, political identity, and so forth. We are members of a community that we did not want to join, but we can be very grateful for its existence. We are bound to each other during active treatment and in the posttreatment stage, existing as marginal people stuck between the worlds of the sick and the well. I would also argue that we are forever affected by the transition to being a cancer patient (and hopefully to being a cancer survivor) due to the demanding rites of passage associated with the diagnosis and treatment of cancer.

My Support Experiences

As noted earlier, I have come to genuinely care about the intimate strangers in my virtual cancer-support communities. @ThanksCancer has provided a forum where I can vent my fears, seek advice, laugh, and get support when needed. Even though I am limited in the length of my posts, I have shared more personal information about my cancer experience with these "strangers," of whom I know only their Twitter/X names, their profile descriptions, and whatever other details/pictures they have shared in their posts, than I have shared with even some of my closest friends.

I have asked for and received nonjudgmental support when I am scared before my checkup dates and/or before blood work and scans. No one on @ThanksCancer tells me that I am being irrational or asks me when I am going to "get past" the experience. They send hugs and then ask how everything went.

We can share information and ask questions of each other that we find hard to ask our oncologists after treatment, such as how many people are suffering lingering neuropathy or muscle cramping and whether anyone has any advice or strategies on how to manage it.

But despite all these benefits, not surprisingly, since this community includes current and former cancer patients, not everyone survives. Since joining @ThanksCancer almost three years ago, I have fiercely wept for a number of community members who did not survive. Their posts became an expected and anticipated part of my online cancer community conversations—they were intimate voices in our collective narrative—and others in the community and I have profoundly felt their silence. But also not surprisingly, new voices join, and as I travel further along my own five-year posttreatment journey, I can provide some advice from my particular vantage point, while those who are even further along their journey than I am continue to provide me guidance.

Returning to Work and Then,
the Pandemic

I returned to full-time teaching in the 2020 spring semester. My hair had started growing back, but at this point, I looked like I was sporting a very edgy buzz cut. It felt magnificent to be back at work, interacting with my colleagues and with the students. I was managing significant fatigue, but the adrenaline rush I regularly felt right before entering the classroom got me through some of the hardest bouts of exhaustion. I was also finally starting to enjoy the taste of coffee again.

That spring semester, I was teaching two sections of introductory sociology and one section of my course Bioethics: A Sociological Perspective. This is how I describe this course on my syllabus:

> Our cultural concept of what defines a "human being," and what defines both normal and desired life experiences, impacts not only the practice of medicine, but also our pursuit of new medical technologies. And once those technologies are created, they may in turn impact our experience and change previous expectations and understandings. . . . In this class, we will explore how wider cultural forces impact the development of medical technologies, and how once a technology exists, society must decide how to use it and encourage or restrict access. The practice of medicine and science does not occur in some objective, rational bubble, but our medical institutions are interwoven within and greatly impacted by wider social norms, by

our political and economic institutions, by power struggles, and by the ever-changing definition of what it means to be a "human being" at different points and time in human history.

Prior to beginning the bioethics class that semester, I had not really reflected on how the experience of teaching this particular class was about to be forever changed by my recent experience with lymphoma. Many of the questions I raise in the class and analyze from bioethical and sociological perspectives were now not fundamentally theoretical questions that I had contemplated as they referred to populations I had studied; they were core questions I had faced myself and knew that I would continue to face going forward.

For example, we talk about the cost of care in the United States and how much money we spend during an individual's last year of life. The estimates can vary based on how this question is tackled, but Karolos Arapakis et al. have found that dying "is expensive in America. Healthcare expenditures from all payors (public and private) total $80,000 in the last 12 months of life and $155,000 in the last 3 years."[1] About one-quarter of all Medicare spending is spent on people in their last year of life.[2] In my course, we discuss the ethicality and rationality of spending these resources during the last year versus investing more resources in younger cohorts. We ask this question in the context of American culture, in the name of advancing knowledge, and in contemplation of what we owe people for their lifetime of participation in society. In conjunction with this analysis, we wrestle with John Hardwig's article "Is There a Duty to Die?"[3] Do we all, despite our desire to live even one more year, owe it to everyone to refuse any more efforts to keep us alive? Can we decide that we have eaten all the apples we should ever eat and leave the rest for others?

The entire process of pursuing my diagnosis and of my treatment was unquestionably expensive. Anyone who has ever reviewed their "Explanation of Benefits" documents from their insurance providers has likely noticed that what a provider charges for a service and what the health plan agrees to pay is often significantly different—a difference inexplicable to those not in the business. But let us look at two examples in my case.

The total cost of my bone biopsy was $54,413.44. This amount included $11,585.00 for the operating room service. Of the total, $50,728.79 was not billable to me, and my insurance company paid $3,684.65. One of my outpatient R-CHOP infusions cost $62,787.00. My insurance provider paid HUP $12,335.96. I completed six outpatient infusions, so even just considering what was actually paid (not what was charged), my outpatient treatment cost $74,015.76.

The chances were good (about 70%) that I could successfully complete treatment, so I might argue that I made a rational choice in pursuing care. But was this financial investment in my survival rational in the biggest sense? I have taken comfort throughout my career in thinking that I do my job well—that I have made some difference in people's lives—but what, if anything, did I owe now that I had consumed so many resources? Did I need to become a better professor? A better mother? A better spouse, sibling, neighbor, or friend? My mind raced with all these questions during our class discussions on the cost of healthcare.

The semester began in the middle of January. By February, we had started talking about COVID-19 in our classes. And in March 2020, everyone left campus, and all courses were taught online. I felt like I had just returned, and now I was leaving again.

Strategies for Dealing with the Pandemic

Soon after starting treatment, I became immunocompromised, as the chemotherapy was rapidly diminishing my white blood cell count. As noted earlier, this effect was expected. During treatment, my husband and I established certain routines at home to minimize the possibility of my being exposed to viruses and bacteria. We kept a bottle of hand sanitizer at the front door. We washed our hands incessantly after going out and before any food preparation or consumption. Although we tried to maintain a somewhat-normal routine, I did not attend social events, and I avoided crowds. If my husband attended any social, work, or family gathering, we slept in separate rooms until we were certain that he was not contagious. I went food shopping during off-hours when I knew that I could keep my distance from people. I sterilized my cart. I bought a couple of boxes of masks to wear whenever I just could not avoid crowds, such as when I went into the city for treatment. I only went to one movie during those months—in the middle of the day—and watched it with a mask on! When people came to visit, we talked outside, on my porch (weather permitting), sitting far apart. And all of these precautions worked—I did not "get sick" the entire time I was in treatment.

Just short of three months back in the world, we were all sent home. And now all of us were asked to behave as I had when I was immunocompromised. It was odd to recognize that I "knew what to do" at the beginning of the pandemic when the social-distancing orders went out since I had just had so much practice with all the recommendations. And I even still had supplies—bottles of sanitizer and masks! But I also felt such deep sympathy for everyone, as I knew how the necessary attention to detail to avoid exposure is exhausting and how the lack of interaction with people is isolating and dehumanizing. We are social creatures, and the lack of human touch can be excruciating.

The pandemic did not affect my active treatment, but it did influence my experience of follow-up care, and I am acutely aware of the impact it had on the diagnosis and management of cancer patients generally. One study estimated at least 134,000 missed cancer diagnoses in 2020 in the United States alone, which will result in greater cancer mortality.[4] Other studies suggested that of those who already had confirmed cancer diagnoses at the beginning of the pandemic, 77.5% reported some delay or disruption in their treatment, primarily due to reduction in services by providers because of the extensive demands made by the surge of COVID-19 patients. These included reductions in routine cancer services and number of cancer surgeries, delays in radiotherapy, and delays, reschedules, or cancellations of outpatient visits.[5,6] I counted myself incredibly fortunate to have completed my treatment protocol before the pandemic. My heart breaks for everyone who was told that their treatment would be delayed. How frightening! I found it difficult waiting even fifteen days between my confirmed diagnosis and my first infusion.

A follow-up PET scan that had been scheduled during my first six-month appointment after stopping treatment was canceled as a result of the pandemic. While I completely understood why a PET scan in absence of any obvious indication that my cancer had returned was a non-urgent medical procedure, the possibility of an undetected recurrence at this time raised my anxiety. At this time, I did not suspect that the lymphoma had returned, but I was relying on the scan to reassure my heart that the absence of any obvious symptoms was an accurate representation of what was happening on a cellular level in my body. So soon after treatment, I was still trying to avoid interpreting every ache and pain, every twinge in my shoulder or my hips, as a sign that the cancer was back.

However, I did and still go into Philadelphia for my regular follow-up appointments and blood work. So far, my blood work looks good, except I appear to remain somewhat immunocompromised. Everyone on the floor, including the medical staff and all patients, still mask since unquestionably some people in the waiting room are currently immunocompromised due to treatment.

During my first follow-up visits, I found it extremely hard to walk past the patients who, after their appointments, were waiting to be called back for their infusions. I had to pass them on my way to the checkout desks. As noted in earlier chapters, for every one of my outpatient and inpatient infusions, I was incredibly fortunate to have people with me or visit me. During the first year of the pandemic, patients were no longer allowed to have people accompany them to the appointments or to their infusions at the Abramson Cancer Center. I so wanted to find some way to comfort these patients, whose looks of fatigue and fear were so very familiar, who now had to go it alone during this stage of their treatment because of COVID-19. I trusted that the oncology nurses would take excellent care of them, but who was going to bring them snacks and distract them with silly questions?

At my last medical visit in December 2023, my oncologist was amazed to hear that I had yet to have anything resembling a cold or flu since stopping my treatment. I am completely up-to-date with my COVID-19 vaccines, and I continue to avoid risky encounters and crowded spaces. I remain vigilant since, as noted earlier, I am still somewhat immunocompromised. For the most part, I teach without wearing a mask (except for the first two weeks of the semester, when I know that students are coming from many different places and are likely carrying many different viruses with them). I track the CO_2 levels of the rooms I am in to determine how good the circulation is, and I use a personal and a room air purifier when warranted. Sickness avoidance has become a way of life, especially while I still exist within a five-year posttreatment stage.

Conclusion

As I write this last chapter, in May 2024, I am just six months shy from having my five-year posttreatment medical appointment. If my blood work looks good at that time, I will have reached that coveted five-year posttreatment remission mark, and I will be able to don the "cured" label. I will be able to count myself among the "successfully treated with R-CHOP" patients. I will be a data point in the statistics. Before I schedule that appointment, I have another oncology appointment in less than a month, and I am already feeling the slow and steady increase of my anxiety.

Before my upcoming appointment, I will celebrate my sixtieth birthday! And I have decided to really celebrate this year. My birthday ritual since I was in my late twenties has been to spend the entire day planting in my garden, weather permitting. I get the annual vegetables planted, having already prepared the garden beds. The majority of my garden is filled with native perennials—shrubs, flowers, and herbs—but every year, I always plant some tomatoes, cucumbers, zucchini, and sunflowers. This year, we will also try beets.

My birthday is May 17, and where I live in Pennsylvania, May 15 was for a long time the date when gardeners no longer had to be concerned about the risk of frost. The National Gardening Association reports that as of 2024, the date when there is less than a 10% risk of frost is now April 20—not surprising, given the overall increase in global temperatures.[1] But I still reserve May 17 to do the bulk of my planting, as it really is not until mid-May that the chaos of the spring academic semester has settled enough that I have time to devote to the garden. By my birthday, all my grades have been submitted, graduation has taken place, all May training workshops have been completed, and I can take a moment to catch my breath before summer research activities start.

On May 18, I will celebrate being sixty by first playing pickleball in the early afternoon with my regular pickle crew. I will then host a block party in the early evening for the neighborhood, and I have asked some of my dearest friends and family members to join us. There will be cake, and music, a potluck feast, and undoubtedly much laughter—and reflection and gratitude.

Writing this book has simultaneously been a demanding and enlightening reflection on my cancer experience and, more generally, on the cancer experience in America. I deliberately waited to write Chapter 1, "Pursuing the Diagnosis," until I had written the bulk of the book, as that period of uncertainty and fear was the hardest time to revisit in my narrative. In writing subsequent chapters, I was often distracted by the same focused details that helped me cope during treatment. But many times while writing, a memory would be so powerful as to leave me shedding tears, a reminder, as Bessel van der Kolk and Babette Rothschild have documented, on how intense experiences imprint on our minds and bodies.[2,3]

This concluding chapter provides an opportunity to update readers on some information referenced in earlier chapters. I start with the best reports. I was able to attend my son's white-coat ceremony. He is about to start his fourth year of medical school. I am so proud of his accomplishments, and I am so happy that he will be joining the medical profession. I say this as a very proud mother but also as a professional medical sociologist who has studied physicians!

I was also able to attend my eldest's wedding. The ceremony had to be rescheduled multiple times because of COVID-19, but the day of the ceremony was one of the most perfect days I have ever experienced. They have recently started a master of social work program, where they are specializing in medical trauma!

One of my pups, Audrey, passed away a few months after I finished treatment—she was seventeen. I was so grateful that she stuck around to help get me through treatment. She was a "BDE"—best dog ever. Some months after she passed, we adopted another dog to keep Bowie company—a little deer-faced chihuahua mix that we named Charlie. She is one of the cutest and most feisty dogs—an endless source of entertainment. She is helping Bowie stay young and fit, even though he is now twelve years old (Charlie is now six).

You may recall that Bowie would not leave my side during the period I was pursuing my diagnosis and during active treatment. Since I stopped treatment, he has become much more relaxed. He remains very attached to and protective of me, but he no longer needs to be right next to me all the time. I recognize that sometimes I consciously assess how relaxed he seems, as though perhaps he will detect whether my cancer recurs before any official blood test or scan. If he is not concerned, maybe I can relax as well? As noted before, humans try to find ways to control and predict our tomorrows. When I find myself overly focusing on reading his behavior, I laugh (sometimes slightly maniacally).

I am still adjusting to what now seems to be permanent changes to my body. While most of my food sensitivities faded, I have kept my distaste for most sweet foods. I can consume a few bites but do not enjoy full servings of any sweets. I have no theories. Thank goodness my enjoyment of coffee returned!

All my hair returned, but much thinner than before treatment—that is all the hair except for my random chin hairs, which returned in full force and seem thicker and more numerous now! The somewhat-bald spot on the top of my head remains, which means that I have to be careful when in the sun, especially when I am swimming. My eyelashes still only partially came back—a continuing disappointment, as I occasionally like to wear mascara.

The random muscle cramps and bouts of trigger finger and trigger toe occur less often. I do not know to what degree this lessening is from my figuring out ways to avoid the episodes and to what degree some of my nerves have healed. No matter the reason(s), I am very grateful. Some significant fatigue remains, though it is hard to tell how much of the fatigue is a result of treatment and how much is just from aging.

I finally got my tattoo!

The saddest update is that more members of my online cancer community have passed, while more people recently diagnosed have joined. With every passing, when someone's voice is no longer part of the daily banter and deeper conversations, we are all reminded of how close many of us have been to that moment of nonexistence. We are all reminded that we are mortal. We honor the person, we collectively agree that cancer is terrible, and we hold each other without the burden of being positive and brave. And I cry for people whom I knew only from our virtual community exchanges.

Everyone's future is full of uncertainty, but a cancer experience is a brutal reminder of how much uncertainty there is. My cancer journey is not over, and I recognize that it will never be over, even if I reach the coveted five-year cancer-free mark. While the journey has become and hopefully will continue to become less perilous, I will spend the rest of my life in a body that at one time tried to kill me. I suspect that I will never fully trust my body again, no matter how many years pass. I will remain forever somewhat vigilant.

My experience and this reflection have reinforced my understanding of how the structure of our medical institutions and aspects of our shared culture influence the experience of illness in a society. My hope is that this detailed look at the cancer experience—the good and the bad—can help us collectively identify ways we can reform how we diagnose and treat cancer to improve the experience as much as possible for patients, their families, and the medical teams who treat them and change how we ultimately understand cancer patients' illness narratives. Are there ways we can improve people's access to medical care so that cancers can be caught earlier, lessening society's collective fear of cancer that sometimes contributes to the delay? Can we help improve communication between patients and their caregivers, especially when we recognize how patients' illness states and physical changes challenge the familiar ways we typically present ourselves to the world? Can we better understand that our current cancer metaphors—cancer battles, brave patients, and cancer survivors—instead of empowering patients might unexpectedly silence the expressions of fear and extreme fatigue that they desperately need to communicate as they confront their own mortality? Recent statistics indicate that 41% of American males and 39% of American females will develop cancer over the course of their lifetime.[4] Any reforms will affect many people.

Thinking about my cancer experience and the process of writing this book, do I conclude this chapter with some motivational insights? Do I share some truths that I know at this stage of my journey? I am still betwixt and between, though hopefully getting closer to a recognized and coveted stage.

I will not argue that I am somehow a better person having had this experience, but I will declare that I am incredibly grateful to be alive. I am grateful that I have been able to celebrate some wonderful milestone moments with my children. Having cancer did not make me appreciate life more—I was pretty appreciative before all this happened—but I do pay a bit more attention to beautiful moments. As an avid gardener, I have always celebrated the return of plants every spring. Life bursting from the soil after remaining dormant all winter never ceases to amaze me. But in addition to planting my vegetable garden this year and attending to all my perennials this spring, I will also be planting a sycamore sapling in our yard, a tribute to the future.

As indicated throughout the book, I am also grateful for the countless caring interactions I had and continue to have with members of my medical team and support personnel. The majority of these interactions have illustrated what *should* happen between healthcare professionals and their patients. The depth and authenticity of many of these interactions are models for all of us. In our busy modern lives, we need to take moments to listen to each other's narratives, hold complex truths, and connect. We must recognize that all our narratives are abundantly complex. That is a universal truth of the human condition.

My concluding hope is that I remain in remission so that I continue to have chances to share milestone moments with my children and their partners. To share daily meals with my husband and discuss everything from the changing dynamics of higher education, to the state of world, to where we should take the dogs for a hike. To laugh with my sister and try every cheese Danish and black and white cookie in the tristate area until we can confidently conclude which is the best. To have inspiring discussions with my students and colleagues. To celebrate the milestone moments of my friends' children. To play pickleball as often as I physically can. To swim in the ocean. To watch the catbirds enjoy some raspberries from my garden.

And to continue to advocate for and witness improvements in cancer treatment and in the cancer experience for all patients in America.

NOTES

INTRODUCTION

1. Mills CW. *The Sociological Imagination.* Oxford University Press; 1959.
2. Dr. Fisher reflects on the regimen that changed lymphoma treatment. Fox Chase Cancer Center. September 22, 2017. Accessed July 19, 2018. https://www.foxchase.org/blog/2017-09-22-Ficsher-CHOP-lymphoma

CHAPTER 1

1. Frozen shoulder. OrthoInfo. Reviewed January 2024. Accessed January 14, 2024. https://orthoinfo.aaos.org/en/diseases--conditions/frozen-shoulder
2. Mayo Clinic Staff. Bone metastasis. Mayo Clinic. April 27, 2022. https://www.mayoclinic.org/diseases-conditions/bone-metastasis/symptoms-causes/syc-20370191
3. Shah GL, Rosenberg AS, Jarboe J, Klein A, Cossor F. Incidence and evaluation of incidental abnormal bone marrow signal on magnetic resonance imaging. *Sci. World J.* Published online October 14, 2014. doi:10.1155/2014/380814
4. Moran DE, O'Neill AC, Heffernan EJ, Skehan SJ. Not everything that is hot on a staging bone scan is malignant: a pictorial review of benign causes of increased isotope uptake. *Can Assoc Radiol J.* 2012;63(4):280–288. doi:10.1016/j.carj.2011.02.009
5. PET scan. Cleveland Clinic. Reviewed October 19, 2022. Accessed February 18, 2024. https://my.clevelandclinic.org/health/diagnostics/10123-pet-scan
6. MDsave. Accessed February 18, 2024. https://www.mdsave.com/
7. Kanavos T, Birbas E, Papoudou-Bai A, et al. Primary bone lymphoma: a review of the literature with emphasis on histopathology and histogenesis. *Diseases.* 2023;11(1): 42. doi:10.3390/diseases11010042

CHAPTER 2

1. Parsons T. The sick role and the role of the physician reconsidered. *Milbank Q.* 1975;53(3):257–278. doi:10.2307/3349493

2. Gordon D. For millions of uninsured Americans, the end of 2022 open enrollment is here. *Forbes.* January 15, 2022. https://www.forbes.com/sites/debgordon/2022/01/15 /for-millions-of-uninsured-americans-the-end-of-2022-open-enrollment-is-here/

3. Wilper AP, Woolhandler S, Lasser KE, McCormick D, Bor DH, Himmelstein DU. Health insurance and mortality in US adults. *AJPH.* 2009;99(12):2289–2295. doi:10.2105/AJPH.2008.157685

4. Saad L. More Americans delaying medical treatment due to cost. Gallup. December 9, 2019. https://news.gallup.com/poll/269138/americans-delaying-med ical-treatment-due-cost.aspx?utm_source=alert&utm_medium=email&utm_content =morelink&utm_campaign=syndication

5. Saloner B, Hempstead K, Rhodes K, Polsky D, Pan C, Kenney GM. Most primary care physicians provide appointments, but affordability remains a barrier for the uninsured. *Health Aff.* 2018;(4):627–634. doi:10.1377/hlthaff.2017.0959

6. Woolhandler S, Himmelstein DU. The relationship of health insurance and mortality: is lack of insurance deadly? *Ann Intern Med.* 2017;167(6):424–431. doi:10.7326 /M17-1403

7. Christopher AS, McCormick D, Woolhandler S, Himmelstein DU, Bor DH, Wilper AP. Access to care and chronic disease outcomes among Medicaid-insured persons versus the uninsured. *AJPH.* 2016;106(1):63–69. doi:10.2105/AJPH.2015.302925

8. Institute of Medicine (US) Committee on Health Insurance Status and Its Consequences. *America's Uninsured Crisis: Consequences for Health and Health Care.* National Academies Press; 2009. doi:10.17226/12511

9. Henke RM, Fingar KR, Jiang HJ, Liang L, Gibson TB. Access to obstetric, behavioral health, and surgical inpatient services after hospital mergers in rural areas. *Health Aff.* 2021;40(10):1627–1636. doi:10.1377/hlthaff.2021.00160

10. Kelly C, Hulme C, Farragher T, Clarke G. Are differences in travel time or distance to healthcare for adults in global north countries associated with an impact on health outcomes? A systematic review. *BMJ Open.* 2016;6(11):e013059. doi:10.1136 /bmjopen-2016-013059

11. Taber JM, Leyva B, Persoskie A. Why do people avoid medical care? A qualitative study using national data. *J Gen Intern Med.* 2015;30(3):290–297. doi:10.1007 /s11606-014-3089-1

12. Popik B. Pull yourself up by your bootstraps. The Big Apple. September 9, 2012. https://www.barrypopik.com/index.php/new_york_city/entry/pull_yourself_up _by_your_bootstraps/

13. WLRN Public Media. MLK: a bootless man cannot lift himself by his bootstraps. WLRN. January 17, 2014. https://www.wlrn.org/news/2014-01-17/mlk-a-boot less-man-cannot-lift-himself-by-his-bootstraps

14. Kannan VD, Veazie PJ. Predictors of avoiding medical care and reasons for avoidance behavior. *Med Care.* 2014;52(4):336–345. doi:10.1097/MLR.0000000000000100

15. Zborowski M. *People in Pain.* Jossey-Bass; 1969.

16. Reyes-Gibby CC, Aday LA, Todd KH, Cleeland CS, Anderson KO. Pain in ag-

ing community-dwelling adults in the United States: non-Hispanic Whites, non-Hispanic Blacks, and Hispanics. *J Pain.* 2007;8(1):75–84. doi:10.1016/j.jpain.2006.06.002

17. Meghani S, Polomano RC, Tait RC, Vallerand AH, Anderson KO, Gallagher MG. Advancing a national agenda to eliminate disparities in pain care: directions for health policy, education, practice, and research. *Pain Med.* 2012;13(1):5–28. doi:10.1111/j.1526-4637.2011.01289.x

18. Mossey JM. Defining racial and ethnic disparities in pain management. *Clin Orthop Relat Res.* 2011;469(7):1859–1870. doi:10.1007/s11999-011-1770-9

19. Wyatt R. Pain and ethnicity. *Virtual Mentor.* 2013;15(5):449–454. doi:10.1001/virtualmentor.2013.15.5.pfor1-1305

20. Arias E, Tejada-Vera B, Ahmad F, Kochanek KD. *Vital Statistics Rapid Release: Provisional Life Expectancy Estimates for 2020.* Report No. 015. National Center for Health Statistics. July 2021. https://www.cdc.gov/nchs/data/vsrr/vsrr015-508.pdf

21. PRB. Around the globe, women outlive men. Population Reference Bureau. September 1, 2001. https://www.prb.org/resources/around-the-globe-women-outlive-men/

22. Dattani S, Rodés-Guirao L. Why do women live longer than men? Our World in Data. November 27, 2023. https://ourworldindata.org/why-do-women-live-longer-than-men

23. Doyal L. Sex, gender, and health: the need for a new approach. *BMJ.* 2001;323(7320):1061–1063. doi:10.1136/bmj.323.7320.1061

24. Brett KM, Burt CW. Utilization of ambulatory medical care by women: United States, 1997–98. *Vital Health Stat 13.* 2001;(149):1–46. doi:10.1037/e309022005-001

25. Almost 90% of men/women globally are biased against women. United Nations Development Programme. March 5, 2020. https://www.undp.org/press-releases/almost-90-men/women-globally-are-biased-against-women

26. Moore C. Cost factors that affect women's health. Healthgrades. Updated on March 24, 2023. https://resources.healthgrades.com/right-care/patient-advocate/cost-factors-that-affect-female-health-tips-for-women-to-make-healthcare-more-affordable

27. Samulowitz A, Gremyr I, Eriksson E, Hensing G. "Brave men" and "emotional women": a theory-guided literature review on gender bias in health care and gendered norms towards patients with chronic pain. *Pain Res Manag.* 2018;2018:6358624. doi:10.1155/2018/6358624

28. Wesolowicz DM, Clark JF, Boissoneault J, Robinson ME. The roles of gender and profession on gender role expectations of pain in health care professionals. *J Pain Res.* 2018;11:1121–1128. doi:10.2147/JPR.S162123

29. Westergaard D, Clark JF, Boissoneault J, Robinson ME. Population-wide analysis of differences in disease progression patterns in men and women. *Nat. Commun.* 2019;10(666). doi:10.1038/s41467-019-08475-9

30. Reuters. Women are diagnosed years later than men for same diseases, study finds. NBC News. March 25, 2019. https://www.nbcnews.com/health/health-news/women-are-diagnosed-years-later-men-same-diseases-study-finds-n987216

31. Villines Z. What to know about gender bias in healthcare. MedicalNewsToday. October 25, 2021. https://www.medicalnewstoday.com/articles/gender-bias-in-healthcare

32. Kish JK, Yu M, Percy-Laurry A, Altekruse SF. Racial and ethnic disparities in cancer survival by neighborhood socioeconomic status in Surveillance, Epidemiology,

and End Results (SEER) Registries. *J Natl Cancer Inst Monogr.* 2014;2014(49):236–243. doi:10.1093/jncimonographs/lgu020

33. Morris DB. *Illness and Culture in the Postmodern Age.* University of California Press; 2023.

34. Rae SB. On the connection between sickness and sin: a commentary. *Christ Bioeth.* 2006;12(2):151–156. doi:10.1080/13803600600805310

35. Bury M. Illness narratives: fact or fiction? *Sociol Health Illn.* 2001;23(3):263–285. doi:10.1111/1467-9566.00252

36. Kushner HS. *When Bad Things Happen to Good People.* Anchor; 2004.

37. O'Connell VA. When a child has cancer: protecting children from a toxic world. In: Casper MJ, ed. *Synthetic Planet: Chemical Politics and the Hazards of Modern Life.* Routledge; 2003:111–129.

38. Three Mile Island accident. World Nuclear Association. Updated October 11, 2022. Accessed November 22, 2024. https://world-nuclear.org/information-library /safety-and-security/safety-of-plants/three-mile-island-accident

39. Fallon S. Air pollution in New Jersey is so bad it could be dangerous to your health to breathe. NorthJersey.com. April 18, 2018. https://www.northjersey.com /story/news/environment/2018/04/18/new-jerseys-air-among-worst-nation/521041002/

40. Key statistics for lung cancer. American Cancer Society. Revised January 16, 2025. Accessed November 22, 2024. https://www.cancer.org/cancer/types/lung-can cer/about/key-statistics.html

41. Minkler M. Personal responsibility for health? A review of the arguments and the evidence at century's end. *Health Educ Behav.* 1999;26(1):121–140. doi:10 .1177/109019819902600110

42. Friesen P. Personal responsibility within health policy: unethical and ineffective. *J Med Ethics.* 2018;44(1):53–58. doi:10.1136/medethics-2016-103478

43. Schroeder HA, Tipton IH. The human body burden of lead. *Arch Environ Health.* 1968;17(6):965–978. doi:10.1080/00039896.1968.10665354

44. James W, Jia C, Kedia S. Uneven magnitude of disparities in cancer risks from air toxins. *Int J Environ Res Public Health.* 2012;9(12):4365–4385. doi:10.3390/ijerph 9124365

45. Exposome and exposomics. National Institute for Occupational Safety and Health (NIOSH). April 21, 2014. https://archive.cdc.gov/www_cdc_gov/niosh/to pics/exposome/default.html

46. Holden E. Is modern life poisoning me? I took the tests to find out. *Guardian.* May 22, 2019. https://www.theguardian.com/us-news/2019/may/22/is-modern-life -poisoning-me-i-took-the-tests-to-find-out

47. Hughes C, French C. Medicine and magic. *BMJ.* 2002;324:0205132. doi:10 .1136/sbmj.0205132

48. Kim C, Prabhu AV, Hansberry DR, Agarwal N, Heron DE, Beriwal S. Digital era of mobile communications and smartphones: a novel analysis of patient comprehension of cancer-related information available through mobile applications. *Cancer Invest.* 2019;37(3):127–133. doi:10.1080/07357907.2019.1572760

49. Friedman DB, Hoffman-Goetz L. A systematic review of readability and comprehension instruments used for print and web-based cancer information. *Health Educ Behav.* 2006;33(3):352–373. doi:10.1177/1090198105277329

50. Chapman K, Abraham C, Jenkins V, Fallowfield L. Lay understanding of terms used in cancer consultations. *Psychooncology.* 2003;12(6):557–566. doi:10.1002/pon.673

51. Mariotto AB, Noone A-M, Howlader N, et al. Cancer survival: an overview of measures, uses, and interpretation. *J Natl Cancer Inst Monogr.* 2014;2014(49):145–186. doi:10.1093/jncimonographs/lgu024

52. Lobb EA, Butow PN, Kenny DT, Tattersall MH. Communicating prognosis in early breast cancer: do women understand the language used? *Med J Aust.* 1999;171(6):290–294.

53. Siegel RL, Miller KD, Wagle NS, Jemal A. Cancer statistics, 2023. *CA Cancer J Clin.* 2023;73(1):17–48. doi:10.3322/caac.21763

54. Schuell B, Gruenberger T, Kornek GV, et al. Side effects during chemotherapy predict tumour response in advanced colorectal cancer. *Br J Cancer.* 2005;93(7):744–748. doi:10.1038/sj.bjc.6602783

55. Klastersky J, Paesmans M. Response to chemotherapy, quality of life benefits and survival in advanced non-small cell lung cancer: review of literature results. *Lung Cancer.* 2001;34 Suppl 4:S95–S101. doi:10.1016/s0169-5002(01)00383-x

56. Hagerty RG, Butow PN, Ellis PM, et al. Communicating with realism and hope: incurable cancer patients' views on the disclosure of prognosis. *J Clin Oncol.* 2005;23(6):1278–1288. doi:10.1200/JCO.2005.11.138

57. Fox RC. *Experiment Perilous: Physicians and Patients Facing the Unknown.* Free Press; 1959.

58. Zier LS, Sottile PD, Hong SY, Weissfield LA, White DB. Surrogate decision makers' interpretation of prognostic information: a mixed-methods study. *Ann Intern Med.* 2012;156(5):360–366. doi:10.7326/0003-4819-156-5-201203060-00008

59. Blinder VS, Murphy MM, Vahdat LT, et al. Employment after a breast cancer diagnosis: a qualitative study of ethnically diverse urban women. *J Community Health.* 2012;37(4):763–772. doi:10.1007/s10900-011-9509-9

60. Blinder VS, Gany FM. Impact of cancer on employment. *J Clin Oncol.* 2020; 38(4):302–309. doi:10.1200/JCO.19.01856

61. Mehnert A. Employment and work-related issues in cancer survivors. *Crit Rev Oncol Hematol.* 2011;77(2):109–130. doi:10.1016/j.critrevonc.2010.01.004

62. Banegas MP, Guy GP, Jr, de Moor JS, et al. For working-age cancer survivors, medical debt and bankruptcy create financial hardships. *Health Aff (Millwood).* 2016;35(1):54–61. doi:10.1377/hlthaff.2015.0830

63. Ramsey SD, Bansal A, Fedorenko CR, et al. Financial insolvency as a risk factor for early mortality among patients with cancer. *J Clin Oncol.* 2016;34(9):980–986. doi:10.1200/JCO.2015.64.6620

64. Gilligan AM, Alberts DS, Roe DJ, Skrepnek GH. Death or debt? National estimates of financial toxicity in persons with newly-diagnosed cancer. *Am J Med.* 2018;131(10):1187–1199.e5. doi:10.1016/j.amjmed.2018.05.020

65. Altice CK, Banegas MP, Tucker-Seeley RD, Yabroff KR. Financial hardships experienced by cancer survivors: a systematic review. *J Natl Cancer Inst.* 2016; 109(2):djw205. doi:10.1093/jnci/djw205

66. Ellis L, Canchola AJ, Spiegel D, Ladabaum U, Haile R, Gomez SL. Trends in cancer survival by health insurance status in California from 1997 to 2014. *JAMA Oncol.* 2018;4(3):317–323. doi:10.1001/jamaoncol.2017.3846

67. Prüss A, Kay D, Fewtrell L, Bartram J. Estimating the burden of disease from water, sanitation, and hygiene at a global level. *Environ Health Perspect.* 2002;110(5):537–542. doi:10.1289/ehp.110-1240845

68. Sullivan DH. The role of nutrition in increased morbidity and mortality. *Clin Geriatr Med.* 1995;(4):661–674.

69. Barrow SM, Herman DB, Córdova P, Struening EL. Mortality among homeless shelter residents in New York City. *Am J Public Health.* 1999;89(4):529–534. doi:10.2105/ajph.89.4.529

70. Gundersen C, Ziliak JP. Food insecurity and health outcomes. *Health Aff.* 2015;34(11). doi:10.1377/hlthaff.2015.0645

71. McDougall JA, Anderson J, Jaffe SA, et al. Food insecurity and forgone medical care among cancer survivors. *JCO Oncol Pract.* 2020;16(9):e922–e932. doi:10.1200/JOP.19.00736

72. Zheng Z, Jemal A, Tucker-Seeley R, et al. Worry about daily financial needs and food insecurity among cancer survivors in the United States. *J Natl Compr Canc Netw.* 2020;18(3):315–327. doi:10.6004/jnccn.2019.7359

73. Gany F, Lee T, Ramirez J, et al. Do our patients have enough to eat? Food insecurity among urban low-income cancer patients. *J Health Care Poor Underserved.* 2014;25(3):1153–1168. doi:10.1353/hpu.2014.0145

74. Cormie P, Zopf EM, Zhang X, Schmitz KH. The impact of exercise on cancer mortality, recurrence, and treatment-related adverse effects. *Epidemiol Rev.* 2017;39(1):71–92. doi:10.1093/epirev/mxx007

75. Koshchinsky J, Talen E. Affordable housing and walkable neighborhoods: a national urban analysis. *Cityscape.* 2015;17(2):13–56. https://www.huduser.gov/portal/periodicals/cityscpe/vol17num2/ch1.pdf

CHAPTER 3

1. Signs and symptoms of cancer. American Cancer Society. Revised November 6, 2020. Accessed May 27, 2022. https://www.cancer.org/treatment/understanding-your-diagnosis/signs-and-symptoms-of-cancer.html

2. Symptoms of cancer. National Cancer Institute. Updated May 16, 2019. Accessed May 27, 2022. https://www.cancer.gov/about-cancer/diagnosis-staging/symptoms

3. "Couple," "few," and "several": the (mostly) definitive guide. Merriam-Webster. https://www.merriam-webster.com/words-at-play/couple-few-several-use.

4. King B. 9,096 stars in the sky—is that all? Sky & Telescope. September 17, 2014. https://skyandtelescope.org/astronomy-blogs/how-many-stars-night-sky-09172014/

5. Evans J, Chapple A, Salisbury H, Corrie P, Ziebland S. "It can't be very important because it comes and goes"—patients' accounts of intermittent symptoms preceding a pancreatic cancer diagnosis: a qualitative study. *BMJ Open.* 2014;4(2):e004215. doi:10.1136/bmjopen-2013-004215

6. Mills K, Emery J, Cheung C, Hall N, Birt L, Walter FM. A qualitative exploration of the use of calendar landmarking instruments in cancer symptom research. *BMC Fam Pract.* 2014;15(167). doi:10.1186/s12875-014-0167-8

7. Hansen LA. Challenges patients face in cancer care: implications for the health-care team. *Oncology Pharmacist.* Accessed May 27, 2022. https://www.theoncology pharmacist.com/web-exclusives/14797:top-14797

8. Beauchamp TL, Childress JF. *Principles of Biomedical Ethics.* 7th ed. Oxford University Press; 2013.

9. McCormick TR. Principles of bioethics. UW Medicine Department of Bioethics and Humanities Accessed May 27, 2022. https://depts.washington.edu/bhdept/ethics -medicine/bioethics-topics/articles/principles-bioethics

10. Hippocrates et al. *Of the Epidemics and Historic Epidemics.* LM Publishers; 2020.

11. Ko E, Glazier EM. Is no pain, no gain the best approach to exercise? UCLA Health. July 21, 2021. Accessed May 28, 2022. https://www.uclahealth.org/news/pub lication/no-pain-no-gain-best-approach-exercise

12. Kroner C. No pain, no gain—a myth? UCI Health. April 25, 2019. Accessed May 28, 2022. https://www.ucihealth.org/blog/2019/04/no-pain-no-gain

13. Frenkel M. Refusing treatment. *Oncologist.* 2013;18(5):634–636. doi:10.1634 /theoncologist.2012-0436

14. Huchcroft SA, Snodgrass T. Cancer patients who refuse treatment. *Cancer Causes Control.* 1993;4:179–185. doi:10.1007/BF00051311

15. Puts MTE, Monette J, Girre V, et al. Characteristics of older newly diagnosed cancer patients refusing cancer treatments. *Support Care Cancer.* 2010;18(8):969–974. doi:10.1007/s00520-010-0883-0

16. Schulmeister L. The treatment should not be worse than the disease. *Oncol Nurs News.* 2012;6(3). https://www.oncnursingnews.com/view/the-treatment-should -not-be-worse-than-the-disease

17. Side effects of cancer treatment. National Cancer Institute. Accessed May 29, 2022. https://www.cancer.gov/about-cancer/treatment/side-effects

18. Ondansetron. Medscape. Accessed July 15, 2024. ttps://reference.medscape .com/drug/ondansetron-342052

19. Macquart-Moulin G, Viens P, Bouscary M-L, et al. Discordance between physi-cians' estimations and breast cancer patients' self-assessment of side-effects of chemo-therapy: an issue for quality of care. *Br J Cancer.* 1997;76(12):1640–1645. doi:10.1038 /bjc.1997.610

20. Krok-Schoen JL, Fernandez K, Unzeitig GW, Rubio G, Paskett ED, Post DM. Hispanic breast cancer patients' symptom experience and patient-physician communication during chemotherapy. *Support Care Cancer.* 2019;27(2):697–704. doi:10.1007/s00520-018-4375-y

21. Bevan JL, Pecchioni LL. Understanding the impact of family caregiver can-cer literacy on patient health outcomes. *Patient Educ Couns.* 2008;71(3):356–364. doi:10.1016/j.pec.2008.02.022

22. Thompson T, Ketcher D, Gray TF, Kent EE. The Dyadic Cancer Outcomes Framework: a general framework of the effects of cancer on patients and informal care-givers. *Soc Sci Med.* 2021;287:114357. doi:10.1016/j.socscimed.2021.114357

23. Wolpe PR. The triumph of autonomy in American bioethics: a sociological view. In: DeVries R, Subedi J, eds. *Bioethics and Society: Constructing the Ethical Enter-prise.* Prentice Hall; 1998:38–59.

24. Winlow H. Darwinism and social Darwinism. In: Kitchen R, Thrift N, ed. *International Encyclopedia of Human Geography*. 2nd ed. Elsevier; 2020:149–158. doi:10.1016/b978-0-08-102295-5.10249-5

25. Mills CW. *The Sociological Imagination*. Oxford University Press; 1959.

26. Jennings B. Reconceptualizing autonomy: a relational turn in bioethics. *Hastings Cent Rep*. 2016;46(3):11–16. doi:10.1002/hast.544

27. Mackenzie C, Stoljar N. *Relational Autonomy*. Oxford University Press; 2000.

28. Ho A. Relational autonomy or undue pressure? Family's role in medical decision-making. *Scand J Caring Sci*. 2008;22(1):128–135. doi:10.1111/j.1471-6712.2007.00561.x

29. Walter JK, Ross LF. Relational autonomy: moving beyond the limits of isolated individualism. *Pediatrics*. 2014;133(Supplement_1):S16–S23. doi:10.1542/peds.2013-3608d

30. Adult literacy in the United States. National Center for Education Statistics. July 2019. Accessed June 7, 2022. https://nces.ed.gov/pubs2019/2019179/index.asp

31. Nathan JP, Vider E. The package insert. U.S. Pharmacist. May 15, 2015. https://www.uspharmacist.com/article/the-package-insert

32. Tauber A. Causation and the learned-intermediary doctrine. Drug & Device Law. June 3, 2021. https://www.druganddevicelawblog.com/2021/06/causation-and-the-learned-intermediary-doctrine.html#:~:text=Under%20the%20learned%2Dintermediary%20doctrine,to%20his%20or%20her%20patients

33. Guidance for industry: labeling for human prescription drug and biological products—implementing the PLR content and format requirements. U.S. Food & Drug Administration. February 2013. Accessed January 8, 2025. https://www.fda.gov/downloads/Drugs/GuidanceComplianceRegulatoryInformation/Guidances/ucm075082.pdf

34. R-CHOP. National Cancer Institute. September 18, 2009. Updated May 10, 2023. Accessed June 1, 2022. https://www.cancer.gov/about-cancer/treatment/drugs/r-chop

35. Bonvissuto D. What is a chemo port? WebMD. August 2, 2022. https://www.webmd.com/cancer/what-is-chemo-port

36. PowerPortTM Implantable Port. BD. Accessed August 15, 2024. https://www.bd.com/en-us/products-and-solutions/products/product-page.1759601

37. Spataro J. The real history of black and white cookies. VICE. May 4, 2018. Accessed June 19, 2022. https://www.vice.com/en/article/pax7gg/the-real-history-of-black-and-white-cookies

38. Nyquist J. *The Questions Book*. Publisher unknown; 2019. https://joenyquist.com/thequestionsbook

CHAPTER 4

1. Bateman K. How the pixie cut evolved into today's biggest beauty statement. *Vogue*. April 27, 2021. https://www.vogue.com/article/history-of-the-pixie-cut

2. Merton RK. *Social Theory and Social Structure*. Simon and Schuster; 1962.

3. Goffman E. *Asylums: Essays on the Social Situation of Mental Patients and Other Inmates*. Anchor Books / Doubleday; 1961.

4. Misra R, McKean M. College students' academic stress and its relation to their anxiety, time management, and leisure satisfaction. *Am J Health Stud.* 2000;16(1):41–51.

5. PBS NewsHour YouTube page. The chaos and fog of the first night of Marine Corps boot camp. December 8, 2016. https://www.youtube.com/watch?v=yPK6qlpJ_ug

6. DeFilippis EM. Hidden beneath the hospital gown. *New York Times.* February 18, 2020. https://www.nytimes.com/2020/02/18/well/live/patients-hospital-gowns -doctors.html

7. Goffman E. *The Presentation of Self in Everyday Life.* Anchor; 1956.

8. Shakespeare W. *As You Like It*, act II, scene VII [All the world's a stage]. Poets .org. https://poets.org/poem/you-it-act-ii-scene-vii-all-worlds-stage

9. Mead GH. *Mind, Self, and Society.* University of Chicago Press; 2015.

10. Cooley CH. *Two Major Works.* Free Press; 1909.

11. Brewster K. Beyond classic symbolic interactionism: towards an intersectional reading of George H. Mead's "Mind, Self, and Society." Round table at: American Sociological Association Research Conference; August 2013; New York.

12. Shaffer LS. From mirror self-recognition to the looking-glass self: exploring the Justification Hypothesis. *J Clin Psychol.* 2005;61(1):47–65. doi:10.1002/jclp .20090

13. Topo P, Iltanen-Tähkävuori S. Scripting patienthood with patient clothing. *Soc Sci Med.* 2010;70(11):1682–1689. doi:10.1016/j.socscimed.2010.01.050

14. Bergbom I, Pettersson M, Mattsson E. Patient clothing—practical solution or means of imposing anonymity? *J Hosp Med Manage.* 2017;3(3):22. doi:10.4172/2471 -9781.100041

15. Henry Ford Health Staff. A surprising side effect of cancer treatment? Loss of smell and taste. Henry Ford Health. April 29, 2021. Accessed July 5, 2022. https:// www.henryford.com/blog/2021/04/chemotherapy-loss-of-smell-and-taste

16. Hong JH, Omur-Ozbek P, Stanek BT, et al. Taste and odor abnormalities in cancer patients. *J Support Oncol.* 2009;7(2):58–65.

17. wabbly. Chemical smell post chemo. Blood Cancer UK. February 28, 2019. https://forum.bloodcancer.org.uk/t/chemical-smell-post-chemo/1301

18. Georgia. Chemo smell and what to do about it. Caregiver-Aid. August 3, 2020. Accessed July 2022. https://www.caregiver-aid.com/chemo-smell/

19. Khazan O. How often people in various countries shower. *The Atlantic.* February 17, 2015. https://www.theatlantic.com/health/archive/2015/02/how-often-people -in-various-countries-shower/385470/

20. Statista Research Department. U.S. population: do you use moisturizers / creams / lotions? Statista. February 5, 2024. Accessed August 15, 2024. https://www.statista .com/statistics/276408/us-households-usage-of-moisturizers-creams-and-lotions/

21. McGregor J. Less deodorant, fewer showers, no makeup: the nine extra minutes some Americans sneak by working remote. *Forbes.* February 2, 2022. https://www .forbes.com/sites/jenamcgregor/2022/02/02/less-deodorant-fewer-showers-no-makeup -the-nine-extra-minutes-some-americans-sneak-by-working-remote/?sh=25de5fa15567

22. Everts S. How advertisers convinced Americans they smelled bad. *Smithsonian Magazine.* August 2, 2012. https://www.smithsonianmag.com/history/how-advertisers-convinced-americans-they-smelled-bad-12552404/

23. Ashenburg K. *The Dirt on Clean.* North Point Press; 2014.

24. Penttila N. Ah, sweet skunk! Why we like or dislike what we smell. Dana Foundation. October 1, 2001. https://www.dana.org/article/ah-sweet-skunk-why-we-like-or-dislike-what-we-smell/

25. Pazzaglia M. Body and odors: not just molecules, after all. *Curr Dir Psychol Sci.* 2015;24(4):329–333. doi:10.1177/0963721415575329

26. Fried MP. Overview of smell and taste disorders. Merck Manual Consumer Version. September 9, 2021. Modified September 2023. https://www.merckmanuals.com/home/ear,-nose,-and-throat-disorders/symptoms-of-nose-and-throat-disorders/overview-of-smell-and-taste-disorders

27. Locher JL, Yoels WC, Maurer D, van Ells J. Comfort foods: an exploratory journey into the social and emotional significance of food. *Food Foodw.* 2005;13(4):273–297. doi:10.1080/07409710500334509

28. McQuestion M, Fitch M, Howell D. The changed meaning of food: physical, social and emotional loss for patients having received radiation treatment for head and neck cancer. *Eur J Oncol Nurs.* 2011;15(2):145–151. doi:10.1016/j.ejon.2010.07.006

29. Mayo Clinic Staff. Keratosis pilaris. Mayo Clinic. January 30, 2021. Updated October 23, 2024. https://www.mayoclinic.org/diseases-conditions/keratosis-pilaris/symptoms-causes/syc-20351149

30. Alai AN. Keratosis pilaris. Medscape. October 15, 2020. Updated May 12, 2022. https://www.medscape.com/answers/1070651-4630/what-is-the-global-prevalence-of-keratosis-pilaris-kp#:~:text=Keratosis%20pilaris%20affects%2050%2D80,other%20relationship%20to%20keratosis%20pilaris

31. Anthony K. Understanding keratosis pilaris (chicken skin). Healthline. July 6, 2022. Updated November 22, 2023. https://www.healthline.com/health/keratosis-pilaris

32. Charmaz K. Loss of self: a fundamental form of suffering in the chronically ill. *Sociol Health Illn.* 1983;5(2):168–195. doi:10.1111/1467-9566.ep10491512

CHAPTER 5

1. Types of cancer treatment. National Cancer Institute. Accessed July 21, 2022. https://www.cancer.gov/about-cancer/treatment/types

2. Drugs approved for different types of cancer. National Cancer Institute. Accessed July 21, 2022. https://www.cancer.gov/about-cancer/treatment/drugs/cancer-type

3. A to Z list of cancer drugs. National Cancer Institute. Accessed July 21, 2022. https://www.cancer.gov/about-cancer/treatment/drugs

4. Nunez K. How long does chemotherapy take? Healthline. April 13, 2021. https://www.healthline.com/health/cancer/how-long-is-chemotherapy

5. Weaver CH. Frequently asked questions about the role of maintenance therapy in cancer. CancerConnect. October 3, 2020. Updated April 29, 2024. https://news.cancerconnect.com/treatment-care/frequently-asked-questions-about-the-role-of-maintenance-therapy-in-cancer

6. Goode WJ. A theory of role strain. *Am Sociol Rev.* 1960;25(4):483–496. doi:10.2307/2092933

7. Levinson H. Book review: *Organizational Stress: Studies in Role Conflict and Ambiguity. Adm Sci Q.* 1965;10(1, theme issue):125–129. doi:10.2307/2391654

8. Watanabe T, Yagata H, Saito M, et al. A multicenter survey of temporal changes in chemotherapy-induced hair loss in breast cancer patients. *PLoS One.* 2019;14(1): e0208118. doi:10.1371/journal.pone.0208118

9. Marks SR. Multiple roles and role strain: some notes on human energy, time and commitment. *Am Sociol Rev.* 1977;42(6):921–936. doi:10.2307/2094577

10. Bower JE. Cancer-related fatigue—mechanisms, risk factors, and treatments. *Nat Rev Clin Oncol.* 2014;11(10):597–609. doi:10.1038/nrclinonc.2014.127

11. Lawrence DP, Kupelnick B, Miller K, Devine D, Lau J. Evidence report on the occurrence, assessment, and treatment of fatigue in cancer patients. *J Natl Cancer Inst Monogr.* 2004:2004(32):40–50. doi:10.1093/jncimonographs/lgh027

12. Mayo Clinic Staff. Cancer fatigue: why it occurs and how to cope. Mayo Clinic. July 12, 2022. Updated September 10, 2024. https://www.mayoclinic.org/diseases-conditions/cancer/in-depth/cancer-fatigue/art-20047709

13. John Heinz National Wildlife Refuge at Tinicum. U.S. Fish & Wildlife Service. Accessed August 15, 2024. https://www.fws.gov/refuge/john-heinz-tinicum

CHAPTER 6

1. Friedson E. *Professional Powers.* University of Chicago Press; 1986.

2. Kowarski I. How to fulfill med school admission requirements. *U.S. News & World Report.* August 25, 2022. https://www.usnews.com/education/best-graduate-schools/top-medical-schools/articles/how-to-make-sure-you-fulfill-medical-school-requirements-for-admission#:~:text=The%20most%20important%20requirement%20for,overemphasize%20extracurricular%20activities%2C%2

3. Youngclause J, Roskovennsky L. An updated look at the economic diversity of U.S. medical students. *AAMC Analysis in Brief.* 2018;18(5). Accessed October 3, 2022. https://www.aamc.org/data-reports/analysis-brief/report/updated-look-economic-diversity-us-medical-students

4. Figure 2. Percentage of applicants to U.S. Medical Schools by Race/Ethnicity (alone), academic year 2018–2019. AAMC. March 19, 2019. Accessed October 3, 2022. https://www.aamc.org/data-reports/workforce/interactive-data/figure-2-percentage-applicants-us-medical-schools-race/ethnicity-alone-academic-year-2018-2019

5. QuickFacts: United States. United States Census Bureau. Accessed October 3, 2022. https://www.census.gov/quickfacts/fact/table/US/PST045221

6. Alpert JS, Frishman WH. The most important qualities for the good doctor. *Am J Med.* 2021;134(7):825–826. doi:10.1016/j.amjmed.2020.11.002

7. Paulas R. Why are so many surgeons assholes? *Pacific Standard.* July 20, 2015. https://psmag.com/social-justice/why-is-my-surgeon-acting-like-biff-from-back-to-the-future

8. Hughes KA. This is exactly why surgeons are so fragile. All of them. KevinMD.com. January 23, 2015. https://www.kevinmd.com/2015/01/exactly-surgeons-fragile.html

9. Peterson M. *What Makes a Good Doctor?: The Personal Qualities That Relate to Patient Satisfaction.* Thesis. College of Saint Benedict/Saint John's University; 2011. https://digitalcommons.csbsju.edu/honors_theses/119

10. Jagosh J, Boudreau JD, Steinert Y, MacDonald ME, Ingram L. The importance of physician listening from the patients' perspective: enhancing diagnosis, heal-

ing, and the doctor–patient relationship. *Patient Educ Couns.* 2011;85(3):369–374. doi:10.1016/j.pec.2011.01.028

11. Coulter A. Patients' views of the good doctor. *BMJ.* 2002;325(7366):668–669. doi:10.1136/bmj.325.7366.668

12. Vermeire E, Hearnshaw H, Van Royen P, Denekens J. Patient adherence to treatment: three decades of research. A comprehensive review. *J Clin Pharm Ther.* 2002;26(5):331–342. doi:10.1046/j.1365-2710.2001.00363.x

13. Viswanathan M, Golin CE, Jones CD, et al. Interventions to improve adherence to self-administered medications for chronic diseases in the United States: a systematic review. *Ann Intern Med.* 2012;157(11):785. doi:10.7326/0003-4819-157-11-201212040 -00538

14. Morris LS, Schulz RM. Patient compliance—an overview. *J Clin Pharm Ther.* 1992;17(5):283–295. doi:10.1111/j.1365-2710.1992.tb01306.x

15. Parsons T. The sick role and the role of the physician reconsidered. *Milbank Q.* 1975;53(3):257–278. doi:10.2307/3349493

16. Sointu E. "Good" patient/"bad" patient: clinical learning and the entrenching of inequality. *Sociol Health Illn.* 2016;39(1):63–77. doi:10.1111/1467-9566.12487

17. Aronson L. "Good" patients and "difficult" patients—rethinking our definitions. *N Engl J Med.* 2013;369(9):796–797. doi:10.1056/nejmp1303057

18. Cosentino BW. How and why to be a good patient. Next Avenue. July 27, 2022. https://www.nextavenue.org/how-and-why-to-be-a-good-patient/

19. Schnabel D. 21 tips for patients on how to be good patients: from health care professionals. GomerBlog. March 7, 2015. https://gomerblog.com/2015/03/tips-for -patients/

20. Avitzur O. 5 steps to becoming a great patient. *Consumer Reports.* April 2014. Accessed October 5, 2022. https://www.consumerreports.org/cro/2014/04/5-steps-to -becoming-a-great-patient/index.htm

21. Durkheim E. *The Division of Labor in Society.* Simon and Schuster; 2014.

22. Takeshita J, Wang S, Loren AW, et al. Association of racial/ethnic and gender concordance between patients and physicians with patient experience ratings. *JAMA Netw Open.* 2020;3(11):e2024583. doi:10.1001/jamanetworkopen.2020.24583

23. Huerto R. Minority patients benefit from having minority doctors, but that's a hard match to make. Michigan Medicine, University of Michigan. March 31, 2020. Accessed October 22, 2022. https://labblog.uofmhealth.org/rounds/minority-patients -benefit-from-having-minority-doctors-but-thats-a-hard-match-to-make-0

24. Hill A, Jones D, Woodworth L. Physician-patient race-match reduces patient mortality. *SSRN.* June 26, 2020. Revised August 21, 2020. doi:10.2139/ssrn.3211276

25. Bourdieu P. Cultural reproduction and social reproduction. In: Brown R, ed. *Knowledge, Education, and Cultural Change.* Routledge; 1973:71–112. doi:10.4324/9781 351018142-3

26. Nimmon L, Stenfors-Hayes T. The "handling" of power in the physician-patient encounter: perceptions from experienced physicians. *BMC Med Educ.* 2016;16(114). doi:10.1186/s12909-016-0634-0

27. Quill TE, Brody H. Physician recommendations and patient autonomy: finding a balance between physician power and patient choice. *Ann Intern Med.* 1996;125(9):763–769. doi:10.7326/0003-4819-125-9-199611010-00010

28. Census Bureau releases new educational attainment data. United States Census Bureau. February 24, 2022. https://www.census.gov/newsroom/press-releases/2022/educational-attainment.html

29. Barber N. Should we consider non-compliance a medical error? *BMJ Qual Saf.* 2002;11(1):81–84. doi:10.1136/qhc.11.1.81

30. McKoy JM. Obligation to provide services: a physician-public defender comparison. *AMA J Ethics.* May 2006. Accessed October 22, 2022. https://journalofethics.ama-assn.org/article/obligation-provide-services-physician-public-defender-comparison/2006-05

31. Lorber J. Good patients and problem patients: conformity and deviance in a general hospital. *J Health Soc Behav.* 1975;16(2):213–225. doi:10.2307/2137163

32. Preventing violence against health workers. World Health Organization. Accessed October 23, 2022. https://www.who.int/activities/preventing-violence-against-health-workers

33. Nachreiner NM, Gerberich SG, Ryan AD, McGovern PM. Minnesota nurses' study: perceptions of violence and the work environment. *Ind Health.* 2007;45(5):672–678. doi:10.2486/indhealth.45.672

34. Budd K. Rising violence in the emergency department. AAMC. February 24, 2020. Accessed October 23, 2022. https://www.aamc.org/news-insights/rising-violence-emergency-department

35. Dye TD, Alcantara L, Siddiqi S, et al. Risk of COVID-19-related bullying, harassment and stigma among healthcare workers: an analytical cross-sectional global study. *BMJ Open.* 2020;10(12):e046620. doi:10.1136/bmjopen-2020-046620

36. Harmon GE. Threats, intimidation against doctors and health workers must end. American Medical Association. February 3, 2022. Accessed October 23, 2022. https://www.ama-assn.org/about/leadership/threats-intimidation-against-doctors-and-health-workers-must-end

37. Goffman E. *The Presentation of Self in Everyday Life.* Anchor; 1956.

38. Halford S. Sociologies of space, work and organisation: from fragments to spatial theory. *Sociol Compass.* 2008;2(3):925–943. doi:10.1111/j.1751-9020.2008.00104.x

39. O'Connell VA, Youcha S, Pellegrini V. Physician burnout: the effect of time allotted for a patient visit on physician burnout among OB/GYN physicians. *J Med Pract Manage.* 2009;24(5):300–313.

40. Hinchey SA, Jackson JL. A cohort study assessing difficult patient encounters in a walk-in primary care clinic, predictors and outcomes. *J Gen Intern Med.* 2011;26:588–594. doi:10.1007/s11606-010-1620-6

CHAPTER 7

1. Thomas D. *The Poems of Dylan Thomas.* New Directions Publishing; 2017.

2. Sontag S. *Illness as Metaphor.* Random House Incorporated; 1979.

3. Heederik D, von Mutius E. Does diversity of environmental microbial exposure matter for the occurrence of allergy and asthma? *J Allergy Clin Immunol.* 2012;130(1):44–50. doi:10.1016/j.jaci.2012.01.067

4. Yu W, Yuan X, Xu X, et al. Reduced airway microbiota diversity is associated with elevated allergic respiratory inflammation. *Ann Allergy Asthma Immunol.* 2015;115(1):63–68. doi:10.1016/j.anai.2015.04.025

5. Klass P. Too clean for our children's good? *New York Times.* April 17, 2017. https://www.nytimes.com/2017/04/17/well/family/too-clean-for-our-childrens-good.html

6. Tse K, Horner AA. Allergen tolerance versus the allergic march: the hygiene hypothesis revisited. *Curr Allergy Asthma Rep.* 2008;8:475–483. doi:10.1007/s11882-008-0088-5

7. Renz-Polster H, David MR, Buist AS, et al. Caesarean section delivery and the risk of allergic disorders in childhood. *Clin Exp Allergy.* 2005;35(11):1466–1472. doi:10.1111/j.1365-2222.2005.02356.x

8. Okada H, Kuhn C, Feillet H, Bach J-F. The "hygiene hypothesis" for autoimmune and allergic diseases: an update. *Clin Exp Immunol.* 2010;160(1):1–9. doi:10.1111/j.1365-2249.2010.04139.x

9. Soaps and detergents history. American Cleaning Institute. Accessed December 5, 2022. https://www.cleaninginstitute.org/understanding-products/why-clean/soaps-detergents-history

10. Harris B. Public health, nutrition, and the decline of mortality: the McKeown Thesis revisited. *Soc Hist Med.* 2004;17(3):379–407. doi:10.1093/shm/17.3.379

11. McKeown T, Record RG. Reasons for the decline of mortality in England and Wales during the nineteenth century. *Popul Stud.* 1962;16(2):94–122. doi:10.2307/2173119

12. Frequently asked questions on soap. U.S. Food and Drug Administration. Accessed December 5, 2022. https://www.fda.gov/cosmetics/cosmetic-products/frequently-asked-questions-soap#

13. Bussing-Burks M. Women and post-WWII wages. National Bureau of Economic Research. November 1, 2002. Accessed December 5, 2022. https://www.nber.org/digest/nov02/women-and-post-wwii-wages

14. Jask Media. The history of cleaning. Direct Cleaning Services. November 30, 2018. https://www.directcleaningservicesltd.co.uk/news/the-history-of-cleaning/

15. Ingall M, Renad C, Stebbins S, Real Simple. Cleaning through the ages. CNN. March 26, 2013. https://www.cnn.com/2013/03/26/living/real-simple-cleaning-through-the-ages

16. Associated Press. Win the war on germs. NBC News. October 31, 2003. https://www.nbcnews.com/health/health-news/win-war-germs-flna1c9478757

17. Fighting germs. Nemours KidsHealth. Reviewed June 2023. Accessed December 5, 2022. https://kidshealth.org/en/parents/fighting-germs.html

18. Barker AD, Jordan H. Public attitudes concerning cancer. In: *Holland-Frei Cancer Medicine.* 6th ed. Available at National Center for Biotechnology Information. Accessed December 5, 2022. https://www.ncbi.nlm.nih.gov/books/NBK13445/

19. Clarke JN, Everest MM. Cancer in the mass print media: fear, uncertainty and the medical model. *Soc Sci Med.* 2006;62(10):2591–2600. doi:10.1016/j.socscimed.2005.11.021

20. Vrinten C, McGregor LM, Heinrich M, et al. What do people fear about cancer? A systematic review and meta-synthesis of cancer fears in the general population. *Psychooncology.* 2017;26(8):1070–1079. doi:10.1002/pon.4287

21. Hauser DJ, Schwarz N. The war on prevention II: battle metaphors undermine cancer treatment and prevention and do not increase vigilance. *Health Commun.* 2020;35(13):1698–1704. doi:10.1080/10410236.2019.1663465

22. American Cancer Society Medical and Editorial Content Team. History of cancer treatments: chemotherapy. American Cancer Society. Revised June 12, 2014. Accessed November 22, 2024. https://www.cancer.org/cancer/understanding-cancer /history-of-cancer/cancer-treatment-chemo.html

23. Malm H. Military metaphors and their contribution to the problems of overdiagnosis and overtreatment in the "war" against cancer. *Am J Bioeth*. 2016;16(10):19–21. doi:10.1080/15265161.2016.1214331

24. City of Hope. Far less aggressive approaches are gaining ground for some cancers. City of Hope. November 21, 2018. https://www.cancercenter.com/community /blog/2018/11/far-less-aggressive-approaches-are-gaining-ground-for-some-cancers

25. Jain S. Let's stop talking about "battling cancer." *Scientific American*. January 16, 2020. https://blogs.scientificamerican.com/observations/lets-stop-talking-about -battling-cancer/

26. Cancer mythbusters: the myth that cancer is a "battle." Dana-Farber Cancer Institute. Accessed December 29, 2022. https://www.dana-farber.org/health-library /articles/cancer-mythbusters-the-myth-that-cancer-is-a-battle/

27. Kaiser K. The meaning of the survivor identity for women with breast cancer. *Soc Sci Med*. 2008;67(1):79–87. doi:10.1016/j.socscimed.2008.03.036

28. McCartney M. The fight is on: military metaphors for cancer may harm patients. *BMJ*. 2014;349:g5155. doi:10.1136/bmj.g5155

29. Borchert DM. *The Encyclopedia of Philosophy*. Macmillan Library Reference; 1996.

30. Mehta N. Mind-body dualism: a critique from a health perspective. *Mens Sana Monogr*. 2011;9(1):202–209. doi:10.4103/0973-1229.77436

CHAPTER 8

1. Pinto D. Passing greetings and interactional style: a cross-cultural study of American English and peninsular Spanish. *Multilingua*. 2008;27(4):371–388. doi:10.1515 /multi.2008.017

2. Gesualdi-Gilmore L. "Cancer ghosting" is real: many survivors say friends suddenly disappear after a diagnosis. SurvivorNet. February 22, 2020. https://www.sur vivornet.com/articles/cancer-ghosting-is-real-many-survivors-say-friends-suddenly -disappear-after-a-diagnosis/

3. Tocqueville A. *Democracy in America*. University of Chicago Press; 2002.

4. Gao G. How do Americans stand out from the rest of the world? Pew Research Center. March 12, 2015. Accessed March 8, 2023. https://www.pewresearch.org/fact -tank/2015/03/12/how-do-americans-stand-out-from-the-rest-of-the-world/

5. Keller J. What makes Americans so optimistic? *The Atlantic*. March 25, 2015. https://www.theatlantic.com/politics/archive/2015/03/the-american-ethic-and-the -spirit-of-optimism/388538/

6. Cimons M. Debunking myths about cancer. *Washington Post*. June 10, 2022. https://www.washingtonpost.com/health/2022/06/10/cancer-myths/

7. Bluebond-Langner M. *The Private Worlds of Dying Children*. Princeton University Press; 2020.

8. Traumatic events and post-traumatic stress disorder (PTSD). National Institute of Mental Health. Reviewed February 2025. Accessed March 13, 2023. https://www.nimh.nih.gov/health/topics/post-traumatic-stress-disorder-ptsd

9. How common is PTSD in adults? PTSD: National Center for PTSD. Updated January 15, 2025. Accessed March 13, 2023. https://www.ptsd.va.gov/understand/common/common_adults.asp

10. Miele D, O'Brien EJ. Underdiagnosis of posttraumatic stress disorder in at risk youth. *J Trauma Stress*. 2010;23(5):591–598. doi:10.1002/jts.20572

11. Scheeringa MS. Why PTSD is under-recognized, part I: the Upside Down. *Psychology Today*. February 14, 2018. Accessed March 13, 2023. https://www.psychologytoday.com/us/blog/stress-relief/201802/why-ptsd-is-under-recognized-part-i-the-upside-down

12. Yellowlees PM. An unintended consequence of modern medical practice. Medscape. June 15, 2015. https://www.medscape.com/viewarticle/845533?reg=1&icd=login_success_email_match_norm

13. Parker AM, Sricharoenchai T, Raparla S, Schneck KW, Bienvenu OJ, Needham DM. Posttraumatic stress disorder in critical illness survivors: a metaanalysis. *Crit Care Med*. 2015;43(5):1121–1129. doi:10.1097/ccm.0000000000000882

14. Kangas M, Henry JL, Bryant RA. The course of psychological disorders in the 1st year after cancer diagnosis. *J Consult Clin Psychol*. 2005;73(4):763–768. doi:10.1037/0022-006x.73.4.763

15. Gold JI, Douglas MK, Thomas ML, Elliott JE, Rao SM, Miaskowski C. The relationship between posttraumatic stress disorder, mood states, functional status, and quality of life in oncology outpatients. *J Pain Symptom Manage*. 2012;44(4):520–531. doi:10.1016/j.jpainsymman.2011.10.014

16. Hahn EE, Hays RD, Kahn KL, Litwin MS, Ganz PA. Post-traumatic stress symptoms in cancer survivors: relationship to the impact of cancer scale and other associated risk factors. *Psychooncology*. 2015;24(6):643–652. doi:10.1002/pon.3623

CHAPTER 9

1. Montagu A. *Touching*. HarperCollins; 1986.

2. Ardiel EL, Rankin CH. The importance of touch in development. *Paediatr Child Health*. 2010;15(3):153–156. doi:10.1093/pch/15.3.153

3. Ojanlatva A. Touch as a human tool. *Med Teach*. 1994;16(4):347–353. doi:10.3109/01421599409008272

4. Harmon K. How important is physical contact with your infant? *Scientific American*. May 6, 2010. https://www.scientificamerican.com/article/infant-touch/

5. Hollinger LM. Communicating with the elderly. *J Gerontol Nurs*. 2013;12(3):8–9. doi:10.3928/0098-9134-19860301-05

6. Hollinger LM. Perception of touch in the elderly. *J Gerontol Nurs*. 2013;6(12):741–746. doi:10.3928/0098-9134-19801201-09

7. Weiss SJ. Psychophysiologic effects of caregiver touch on incidence of cardiac dysrhythmia. *Heart Lung*. 1986;15(5):495–505. https://pubmed.ncbi.nlm.nih.gov/3639077/

8. Pérez-Stable EJ, Sabogal F, Otero-Sabogal R, Hiatt RA, McPhee SJ. Misconceptions about cancer among Latinos and Anglos. *JAMA.* 1992;268(22):3219–3223. doi:10.1001/jama.268.22.3219

9. MacInnes P. The handshake is dead. Long live the quick, clean, tender fist bump. *Guardian.* April 22, 2022. https://www.theguardian.com/commentisfree/2022/apr/22/pandemic-fist-bump-barack-obama-covid

10. Linebaugh K, Knutson R. Dr. Anthony Fauci on how life returns to normal. *The Journal.* April 7, 2020. https://www.wsj.com/podcasts/the-journal/dr-anthony-fauci-on-how-life-returns-to-normal/d5754969-7027-431e-89fa-e12788ed9879

11. Oxlund B. An anthropology of the handshake. *Anthropol Now.* 2020;12(1):39–44. doi:10.1080/19428200.2020.1761216

12. Schiffrin D. Handwork as ceremony: the case of the handshake. *Semiotica.* 1974;12(3):189–202. doi:10.1515/semi.1974.12.3.189

13. Chaplin WF, Phillips JB, Brown JD, Clanton NR, Stein JL. Handshaking, gender, personality, and first impressions. *J Pers Soc Psychol.* 2000;79(1):110–117. doi:10.1037/0022-3514.79.1.110

14. Stewart GL, Dustin SL, Barrick MR, Darnold TC. Exploring the handshake in employment interviews. *J Appl Psychol.* 2008;93(5):1139–1146. doi:10.1037/0021-9010.93.5.1139

15. Cohen J. Seven super revealing things your handshake says about you. *Forbes.* June 2, 2015. https://www.forbes.com/sites/jennifercohen/2015/06/02/7-super-revealing-things-your-handshake-says-about-you/?sh=890d67c443da

16. Hitti M. Patients school doctors in manners. CBS News. June 12, 2007. https://www.cbsnews.com/news/patients-school-doctors-in-manners/

17. Lecat P, Dhawan N, Hartung PJ, Gerzina H, Larson R, Konen-Butler C. Improving patient experience by teaching empathic touch and eye gaze: a randomized controlled trial of medical students. *J Patient Exp.* 2020;7(6):1260–1270. doi:10.1177/2374373520916323

18. Bensing JM, Verheul W, van Dulmen AM. Patient anxiety in the medical encounter: a study of verbal and nonverbal communication in general practice. *Health Educ.* 2008;108(5):373–383. doi:10.1108/09654280810899993

19. Cocksedge S, George B, Renwick S, Chew-Graham CA. Touch in primary care consultations: qualitative investigation of doctors' and patients' perceptions. *Br J Gen Pract.* 2013;63(609):e283–e290. doi:10.3399/bjgp13x665251

20. Sointu E. Complementary and alternative medicines, embodied subjectivity and experiences of healing. *Health.* 2013;17(5):530–545. doi:10.1177/1363459312472080

21. Rousseau PC, Blackburn G. The touch of empathy. *J Palliat Med.* 2008;11(10):1299–1300. doi:10.1089/jpm.2008.0174

22. Palpation. MedlinePlus. Reviewed February 2, 2023. Accessed April 15, 2023. https://medlineplus.gov/ency/article/002284.htm

23. Goldiner S. Medicine in the Middle Ages. The Met. January 1, 2012. https://www.metmuseum.org/toah/hd/medm/hd_medm.htm

24. Bottorff JL. The use and meaning of touch in caring for patients with cancer. *Oncol Nurs Forum.* 1993;20(10):1531–1538.

25. Chang SO. The conceptual structure of physical touch in caring. *J Adv Nurs.* 2001;33(6):820–827. doi:10.1046/j.1365-2648.2001.01721.x

26. Leder D, Krucoff MW. The touch that heals: the uses and meanings of touch in the clinical encounter. *J Altern Complement Med.* 2008;14(3):321–327. doi:10.1089 /acm.2007.0717

CHAPTER 10

1. Chabner BA, Fine RL, Allegra CJ, Yeh GW, Curt GA. Cancer chemotherapy: progress and expectations, 1984. *Cancer.* 1984;54(S2):2599–2608. doi:10.1002/1097 -0142(19841201)54:2+<2599::aid-cncr2820541403>3.0.co;2-m

2. Roche B, Clarke PA, Ford D, Shaver SC, Thompson J. High-dose methotrex-ate: nursing considerations for administration and supportive care. *Clin J Oncol Nurs.* 2023;27(1):47–54. doi:10.1188/23.cjon.47-54

3. Our story and our mission. MIB Agents. Accessed May 26, 2023. https://www .mibagents.org/about-us/mission-origin

4. Goffman E. *Asylums: Essays on the Social Situation of Mental Patients and Other Inmates.* Anchor Books / Doubleday; 1961.

5. Capps D. The mortification of the self: Erving Goffman's analysis of the mental hospital. *Pastoral Psychol.* 2016;65:103–126. doi:10.1007/s11089-015-0665-1

6. "A device used to draw blood and give treatments, including intravenous fluids, drugs, or blood transfusions. A thin, flexible tube is inserted into a vein in the upper arm and guided (threaded) into a large vein above the right side of the heart called the superior vena cava. A needle is inserted into a port outside the body to draw blood or give fluids. A PICC may stay in place for weeks or months and helps avoid the need for repeated needle sticks. Also called peripherally inserted central catheter" (PICC, National Cancer Institute, https://www.cancer.gov/publications/dictionaries/cancer-terms/def/picc).

7. Pile KD, Graham GG. Methotrexate. In: Parnham MJ, ed. *Compendium of In-flammatory Diseases.* Springer, Basel; 2016:934–942. doi:10.1007/978-3-7643-8550 -7_47

8. Iftikhar N. What's a normal blood pH and what makes it change? Healthline. August 16, 2019. https://www.healthline.com/health/ph-of-blood

9. Kuznar W. Preventing methotrexate toxicity: know how to use leucovorin, glu-carpidase. *Oncology Pharmacist.* 2013;6(2). Accessed June 8, 2023. https://www.the oncologypharmacist.com/issues/2013/may-2013-vol-6-no-2/15792:preventing-metho trexate-toxicity-know-howtouse-leucovorin

10. Aquaphor ointment creates a semi-occlusive barrier on the skin that allows the outflow of excess fluid and the inflow of oxygen (Aquaphor Healing Ointment: how it works, Aquaphor, January 2017, https://www.aquaphorus.com/specials/how-it-works).

11. Tipton K, Leas BF, Mull NK, et al. *Interventions to Decrease Hospital Length of Stay.* U.S. Agency for Healthcare Research and Quality; 2021. Technical Brief No. 40.

12. Roemer M. *Cancer-Related Hospitalizations for Adults, 2017.* U.S. Agency for Healthcare Research and Quality; 2021. H-CUP Statistical Brief No. 270. www.hcup -us.ahrq.gov/reports/statbriefs/sb270-Cancer-Hospitalizations-Adults-2017.pdf

13. A port ideally needs to be accessed only once during an inpatient stay. After the initial access, the lines can be changed easily.

14. Zerubavel E. *Patterns of Time in Hospital Life*. University of Chicago Press; 1979.

15. Financial and health-related worries keeping Americans up at night, survey shows. American Academy of Sleep Medicine. September 26, 2022. https://aasm.org /financial-and-health-related-worries-keeping-americans-up-at-night-survey-shows/

16. Raypole C. 23 ways to revamp your nighttime routine. Healthline. September 23, 2020. https://www.healthline.com/health/nighttime-routine

17. Mayo Clinic Staff. Sleep Tips: 6 Steps to Better Sleep—Mayo Clinic. Mayo Clinic. May 7, 2022. https://www.mayoclinic.org/healthy-lifestyle/adult-health/in -depth/sleep/art-20048379

18. Morse AM, Bender E. Sleep in hospitalized patients. *Clocks & Sleep*. 2019;1(1): 151–165. doi:10.3390/clockssleep1010014

19. Park MJ, Yoo JH, Cho BW, Kim KT, Jeong W-C, Ha M. Noise in hospital rooms and sleep disturbance in hospitalized medical patients. *Environ Health Toxicol*. 2014;29:e2014006. doi:10.5620/eht.2014.29.e2014006

20. Wesselius HM, van den Ende ES, Alsma J, et al. Quality and quantity of sleep and factors associated with sleep disturbance in hospitalized patients. *JAMA Intern Med*. 2018;178(9):1201–1208. doi:10.1001/jamainternmed.2018.2669

21. Jemisin NK. *The Fifth Season*. Orbit; 2015.

22. Jemisin NK. *The Obelisk Gate*. Orbit; 2016.

23. Hamilton DK. The evidence-based hospital—a case for single-patient rooms. *JAMA Intern Med*. 2019;179(11):1507–1508. doi:10.1001/jamainternmed.2019.2797

24. Office for Civil Rights. HIPAA for professionals. U.S. Department of Health and Human Services. Reviewed Juny 19, 2024. https://www.hhs.gov/hipaa/for-profes sionals/index.html

25. Maltzman JD, Millar LB. Chemotherapy primer: Why? What? And how? Onco-Link. Reviewed August 13, 2010. Accessed July 7, 2023. https://www.oncolink.org/can cer-treatment/cancer-medications/overview/chemotherapy-primer-why-what-and-how#

26. Starr JR. Pregnancy and bone density: what to know. Hospital for Special Surgery. October 15, 2021. Accessed July 7, 2023. https://www.hss.edu/article_pregnancy -bone-density.asp

27. Talking to pregnant women about oral health. Centers for Disease Control and Prevention. Accessed July 7, 2023. https://www.cdc.gov/oral-health/hcp/conversation -tips/talking-to-pregnant-women-about-oral-health.html

28. Upendran A, Gupta R, Geiger Z. Dental infection control. In: *StatPearls* [Internet]. StatPearls Publishing; 2023.

29. What is morphine? Healthdirect. Reviewed May 2023. Accessed July 8, 2023. https://www.healthdirect.gov.au/morphine#what is

30. Central nervous system depressant. National Cancer Institute. Accessed July 8, 2023. https://www.cancer.gov/publications/dictionaries/cancer-terms/def/central -nervous-system-depressant

31. Little B. When cigarette companies used doctors to push smoking. History. September 13, 2018. Updated March 28, 2023. Accessed July 10, 2023. https://www .history.com/news/cigarette-ads-doctors-smoking-endorsement

32. Current guidelines. Office of Disease Prevention and Health Promotion. Accessed July 9, 2023. https://health.gov/our-work/nutrition-physical-activity/physical -activity-guidelines/current-guidelines

33. Exercise or physical activity. National Center for Health Statistics. Reviewed September 24, 2024. Accessed July 9, 2023. https://www.cdc.gov/nchs/fastats/exercise .htm

34. Wendler R. Exercise during cancer treatment: 4 things to know. MD Anderson Cancer Center. October 12, 2022. https://www.mdanderson.org/cancerwise/exercise -during-cancer-treatment--4-things-to-know.h00-159543690.html

35. Roth AJ. Study shows patients are less active after cancer diagnosis. Memorial Sloan Kettering Cancer Center. January 25, 2017. https://www.mskcc.org/news/new -workout-plan-study-shows-patients-are-less-active-after-cancer-diagnosis

36. Ravitch LM. Get on the bandwagon: A Philadelphia sports fan starter glossary. Billy Penn at WHYY. October 25, 2022. https://billypenn.com/2022/10/25/philadel phia-sports-fan-glossary-mascots-catch-phrase/

37. Allen D. Negotiating the role of expert carers on an adult hospital ward. *Sociol Health Illn*. 2000;22(2):149–171. doi:10.1111/1467-9566.00197

38. Strauss AL. *Social Organization of Medical Work*. Transaction Publishers; 1997.

CHAPTER 11

1. Simmel G. The stranger. In: Longhofer W, Winchester D, eds. *Social Theory Rewired*. 3rd ed. Routledge; 2023:446–449. doi:10.4324/9781003320609-57

2. Rubin LB. *Intimate Strangers*. Harper and Row; 1983.

3. Durkheim E. *The Division of Labor in Society*. Simon and Schuster; 2014.

4. Horgan M. Strangers and strangership. *J Intercult Stud*. 2012;33(6):607–622. doi:10.1080/07256868.2012.735110

5. McLemore SD. Simmel's "stranger": a critique of the concept. *Pac Sociol Rev*. 1970;13(2):86–94. doi:10.2307/1388311

6. Hughes EC. *The Sociological Eye*. Routledge; 1971.

7. Schuetz A. The stranger: an essay in social psychology. *Am J Sociol*. 1944;49(6):499–507. doi:10.1086/219472

8. Morgan DHJ. *Rethinking Family Practices*. Palgrave Macmillan UK; 2011. doi:10.1057 /9780230304680

9. Luckow ST. Intimacy among relative strangers: practices of touch and bodily care in new foster care relationships. *Sociol Rev*. 2020;68(1):177–191. doi:10.1177 /0038026119868653

10. Karakayali N. The uses of the stranger: circulation, arbitration, secrecy, and dirt. *Sociol Theory*. 2006;24(4):312–330. doi:10.1111/j.1467-9558.2006.00293.x

11. Watson K. Gallows humor in medicine. *Hastings Cent Rep*. 2011;41(5):37–45. doi:10.1002/j.1552-146x.2011.tb00139.x

12. Shem S. *The House of God*. Penguin; 2010.

13. Wanzer M, Booth-Butterfield M, Booth-Butterfield S. "If we didn't use humor, we'd cry": humorous coping communication in health care settings. *J Health Commun*. 2005;10(2):105–125. doi:10.1080/10810730590915092

14. Piemonte NM, Abreu S. Responding to callous humor in health care. *AMA J Ethics*. 2020;22(7):E608–E614. doi:10.1001/amajethics.2020.608

CHAPTER 12

1. van Gennep A. *The Rites of Passage*. University of Chicago Press; 1966.

2. Bellis MA, Downing J, Ashton JR. Adults at 12? Trends in puberty and their public health consequences. *J Epidemiol Community Health*. 2006;60:910–911. doi:10.1136/jech.2006.049379

3. Allie. A history of bachelor and bachelorette parties. Odyssey. June 14, 2016. https://www.theodysseyonline.com/last-night-of-freedom

4. Mayo Clinic Staff. Cancer diagnosis: 11 tips for coping. Mayo Clinic. September 13, 2022. https://www.mayoclinic.org/diseases-conditions/cancer/in-depth/cancer-diagnosis/art-20044544

5. The hero's journey: explained in 12 steps. Become a Writer Today. December 16, 2020. https://becomeawritertoday.com/heros-journey/

6. MasterClass. Writing 101: what is the hero's journey? 2 hero's journey examples in film. MasterClass. September 3, 2021. https://www.masterclass.com/articles/writing-101-what-is-the-heros-journey

7. 10 movies that follow the hero's journey. Become a Writer Today. January 17, 2023. https://becomeawritertoday.com/movies-that-follow-the-heros-journey/

8. Dapkevičiūtė A, Šapoka V, Martynova E, Pečeliūnas V. Time from symptom onset to diagnosis and treatment among haematological malignancies: influencing factors and associated negative outcomes. *Medicina (Kaunas)*. 2019;55(6):238. doi:10.3390/medicina55060238

9. Klimmek R, Wenzel J. Adaptation of the Illness Trajectory Framework to describe the work of transitional cancer survivorship. *Oncol Nurs Forum*. 2012;39(6):E499–E510. doi:10.1188/12.onf.e499-e510

10. Carr K. *Crazy Sexy Cancer Survivor*. Rowman and Littlefield; 2008.

11. Ehrenreich B. Welcome to Cancerland. *Harper's Magazine*. November 2001. Accessed September 4, 2023. https://harpers.org/archive/2001/11/welcome-to-cancerland/

12. Ehrenreich B. *Bright-Sided*. Macmillan; 2009.

13. Bell K. Remaking the self: trauma, teachable moments, and the biopolitics of cancer survivorship. *Cult Med Psychiatry*. 2012;36:584–600. doi:10.1007/s11013-012-9276-9

14. McBride CM, Emmons KM, Lipkus IM. Understanding the potential of teachable moments: the case of smoking cessation. *Health Educ Res*. 2003;18(2):156–170. doi:10.1093/her/18.2.156

15. del Vecchio Good M-J, Good BJ, Schaffer C, Lind SE. American oncology and the discourse on hope. *Cult Med Psychiatry*. 1990;14:59–79. doi:10.1007/bf00046704

16. Segal J. Cancer isn't the best thing that ever happened to me. *Vancouver Sun*. April 1, 2010.

17. Kahalley LS, Ris MD, Grosshans DR, et al. Comparing intelligence quotient change after treatment with proton versus photon radiation therapy for pediatric brain tumors. *J Clin Oncol*. 2016;34(10):1043–1049. doi:10.1200/jco.2015.62.1383

18. Frank AW. *The Wounded Storyteller*. University of Chicago Press; 2013.

19. Katz A. *After You Ring the Bell . . . 10 Challenges for the Cancer Survivor*. Hygeia Media; 2012.

20. Houtz J. Can Roundup cause cancer? Washington University Department of Environmental and Occupational Health Sciences. February 14, 2019. Accessed September 6, 2023. https://deohs.washington.edu/edge/blog/can-roundup-cause-cancer

21. Cardiotoxicity: cancer treatment and the heart. Cleveland Clinic. Reviewed June 20, 2022. Accessed October 23, 2023. https://my.clevelandclinic.org/health/diseases/16858-chemotherapy--the-heart-cardiotoxicity

22. Mayo Clinic Staff. Peripheral neuropathy. Mayo Clinic. September 2, 2023. https://www.mayoclinic.org/diseases-conditions/peripheral-neuropathy/symptoms-causes/syc-20352061

23. American Cancer Society Medical and Editorial Content Team. Leg cramps. American Cancer Society. Revised March 29, 2024. Accessed October 23, 2023. https://www.cancer.org/cancer/managing-cancer/side-effects/pain/leg-cramps.html

24. Siegal T. Muscle cramps in the cancer patient: causes and treatment. *J Pain Symptom Manage.* 1991;6(2):84–91. doi:10.1016/0885-3924(91)90522-6

25. Buzaglo JS, Miller SM, Kendall J, et al. Evaluation of the efficacy and usability of NCI's *Facing Forward* booklet in the cancer community setting. *J Cancer Surviv.* 2013;7:63–73. doi:10.1007/s11764-012-0245-7

CHAPTER 13

1. Merton RK. Insiders and outsiders: a chapter in the sociology of knowledge (1972). In: Sollors W, ed. *Theories of Ethnicity.* New York University Press; 1996:325–369. doi:10.1007/978-1-349-24984-8_19

2. Book review: *The Marginal Man* by Everett V. Stonequist. *J Educ Sociol.* 1938;11(6, theme issue):381. doi:10.2307/2262260

3. This shared intimacy is not unlike that described by Lily Cho in her article "Intimacy among Strangers." Cho L. Intimacy among strangers: anticipating citizenship in Chinese head tax photographs. *Interventions.* 2013;15(1):10–23. doi:10.1080/1369801x.2013.770996

4. Armes J, Crowe M, Colbourne L, et al. Patients' supportive care needs beyond the end of cancer treatment: a prospective, longitudinal survey. *J Clin Oncol.* 2009;27(36):6172–6179. doi:10.1200/jco.2009.22.5151

5. Harrison JD, Young JM, Price MA, Butow PN, Solomon MJ. What are the unmet supportive care needs of people with cancer? A systematic review. *Support Care Cancer.* 2009;17:1117–1128. doi:10.1007/s00520-009-0615-5

6. Bauman Z. *Modernity and Ambivalence.* John Wiley and Sons; 2013.

7. Horgan M. Strangers and strangership. *J Intercult Stud.* 2012;33(6):607–622. doi:10.1080/07256868.2012.735110

CHAPTER 14

1. Arapakis K, French E, Jones J, McCauley J. How should we fund end-of-life care in the US? *Lancet Reg Health Am.* 2022;15:100359. doi:10.1016/j.lana.2022.100359

2. Jha AK. End-of-life care, not end-of-life spending. JAMA Network. July 13, 2018. https://jamanetwork.com/channels/health-forum/fullarticle/2760146

3. Hardwig J. Is there a duty to die? *Hastings Cent Rep.* 1997;27(2):34–42. doi:10 .2307/3527626

4. Soucheray S. Study estimates 134,000 missed cancer diagnoses in US in 2020. Center for Infectious Disease Research and Policy at the University of Minnesota. February 26, 2024. Accessed February 28, 2024. https://www.cidrap.umn.edu/covid-19 /study-estimates-134000-missed-cancer-diagnoses-us-2020

5. Riera R, Bagattini AM, Pacheco RL, Pachito DV, Roitberg F, Ilbawi A. Delays and disruptions in cancer health care due to COVID-19 pandemic: systematic review. *JCO Glob Oncol.* 2021;7(1):311–323. doi:10.1200/go.20.00639

6. Stone W. Cancer patients face treatment delays during COVID-19. Cancer Health. April 16, 2020. https://www.cancerhealth.com/article/cancer-patients-face -treatment-delays-covid19

CONCLUSION

1. Home page. National Gardening Association. https://garden.org/

2. van der Kolk B. *The Body Keeps the Score.* Penguin Books; 2015.

3. Rothschild B. *The Body Remembers Continuing Education Test: The Psychophysiology of Trauma and Trauma Treatment.* W. W. Norton; 2000.

4. Elflein J. Probability of developing invasive cancer in the U.S. for the period 2017–2019, by gender and age. Statista. March 24, 2024. Accessed May 10, 2024. https://www.statista.com/statistics/268510/probability-of-developing-invasive-cancer -in-the-us-by-gender-and-age/

INDEX

VIRGINIA ADAMS O'CONNELL is Associate Professor and Chair of the Department of Sociology and Anthropology at Moravian University and the author of *Getting Cut: Failing to Survive Surgical Residency Training*.

www.ingramcontent.com/pod-product-compliance
Lightning Source LLC
Chambersburg PA
CBHW022355280326
41935CB00007B/194